This report contains the collective views of an international group of experts and does not necessarily represent the decisions or the stated policy of the United Nations Environment Programme, the International Labour Organisation, or the World Health Organization

Environmental Health Criteria 92

RESMETHRINS — RESMETHRIN BIORESMETHRIN CISRESMETHRIN

Published under the joint sponsorship of the United Nations Environment Programme, the International Labour Organisation, and the World Health Organization

World Health Organization
Geneva, 1989

The International Programme on Chemical Safety (IPCS) is a joint venture of the United Nations Environment Programme, the International Labour Organisation, and the World Health Organization. The main objective of the IPCS is to carry out and disseminate evaluations of the effects of chemicals on human health and the quality of the environment. Supporting activities include the development of epidemiological, experimental laboratory, and risk-assessment methods that could produce internationally comparable results, and the development of manpower in the field of toxicology. Other activities carried out by the IPCS include the development of know-how for coping with chemical accidents, coordination of laboratory testing and epidemiological studies, and promotion of research on the mechanisms of the biological action of chemicals.

ISBN 92 4 154292 6

The designations employed and the presentation of the material in this publication do not imply the expression of any opinion whatsoever on the part of the Secretariat of the World Health Organization concerning the legal status of any country, territory, city or area or of its authorities, or concerning the delimitation of its frontiers or boundaries.

The mention of specific companies or of certain manufacturers' products does not imply that they are endorsed or recommended by the World Health Organization in preference to others of a similar nature that are not mentioned. Errors and omissions excepted, the names of proprietary products are distinguished by initial capital letters.

PRINTED IN FINLAND

Vammalan Kirjapaino Oy

89/8070 — Vammala — 5000

ENVIRONMENTAL HEALTH CRITERIA FOR RESMETHRINS

WHO TASK GROUP ON ENVIRONMENTAL HEALTH CRITERIA FOR ALLETHRINS AND RESMETHRINS

Members

Dr L.A. Albert-Palacios, National Institute of Biological Resources Research, Xalapa, Veracruz, Mexico[a]

Dr V. Benes, Institute of Hygiene and Epidemiology, Prague, Czechoslovakia

Dr A.H. El-Sabae, Faculty of Agriculture, Alexandria University, Alexandria, Egypt

Dr Y. Hayashi, National Institute of Hygienic Sciences, Tokyo, Japan

Dr S. Johnson, US Environmental Protection Agency, Hazard Evaluation Division, Washington DC, USA

Dr S.K. Kashyap, National Institute of Occupational Health, Ahmedabad, India (Vice-Chairman)

Dr J.H. Koeman, Agricultural University, Wageningen, Netherlands[a]

Dr Yu. I. Kundiev, Research Institute of Labour, Hygiene and Occupational Diseases, Kiev, USSR (Chairman)

Dr J.P. Leahey, ICI Agrochemicals Division, Jealotts Hill Research Station, Bracknell, Berkshire, United Kingdom (Rapporteur)

Dr M. Matsuo, Sumitomo Chemical Co. Ltd, Takarazuka Research Center, Takarazuka, Hyogo, Japan

Dr G.U. Oleru, College of Medicine, University of Lagos, Lagos, Nigeria

Observers

Mr J.-M. Pochon, International Group of National Associations of Agrochemical Manufacturers, Brussels, Belgium

Dr L.M. Sasynovitch, Research Institute of Hygiene and Toxicology of Pesticides, Polymers and Plastics, Kiev, USSR

---

[a] Invited but unable to attend.

Secretariat

Dr Z.P. Grigorevskaja, Centre for International Projects, Moscow, USSR

Dr K.W. Jager, International Programme on Chemical Safety, World Health Organization, Geneva, Switzerland (Secretary)

Dr J. Sekizawa, National Institute of Hygienic Sciences, Tokyo, Japan (Rapporteur)

NOTE TO READERS OF THE CRITERIA DOCUMENTS

Every effort has been made to present information in the criteria documents as accurately as possible without unduly delaying their publication. In the interest of all users of the environmental health criteria documents, readers are kindly requested to communicate any errors that may have occurred to the Manager of the International Programme on Chemical Safety, World Health Organization, Geneva, Switzerland, in order that they may be included in corrigenda, which will appear in subsequent volumes.

* * *

A detailed data profile and a legal file can be obtained from the International Register of Potentially Toxic Chemicals, Palais des Nations, 1211 Geneva 10, Switzerland (Telephone no. 7988400 - 7985850).

ENVIRONMENTAL HEALTH CRITERIA FOR RESMETHRINS

A WHO Task Group on Environmental Health Criteria for Allethrins and Resmethrins met in Moscow from 16 to 20 November 1987. The meeting was convened with the financial assistance of the United Nations Environment Programme (UNEP) and was hosted by the Centre for International Projects of the USSR State Committee on Science and Technology. On behalf of the USSR Commission for UNEP (UNEPCOM), Dr M.I. Gunar opened the Meeting and welcomed the participants. Dr K.W. Jager welcomed the participants on behalf of the Heads of the three IPCS cooperating organizations (UNEP/ILO/WHO). The group reviewed and revised the draft Environmental Health Criteria and Health and Safety Guides and made an evaluation of the risks for human health and the environment from exposure to allethrins and resmethrins.

The first drafts of the documents were prepared by Dr J. Miyamoto and Dr M. Matsuo of Sumitomo Chemical Co. Ltd, with the assistance of the staff of the National Institute of Hygienic Sciences, Tokyo, Japan. Dr I. Yamamoto of the Tokyo University of Agriculture and Dr M. Eto of Kyushu University, Japan, assisted in the finalization of the draft.

The second draft was prepared by Dr J. Sekizawa of the National Institute of Hygienic Sciences, Tokyo, incorporating comments received following the circulation of the first draft to the IPCS contact points for Environmental Health Criteria documents.

The help of the Sumitomo Chemical Company Ltd, Japan and Roussel Uclaf, France in making their toxicological proprietary information on allethrins and resmethrins available to the IPCS and the Task Group is gratefully acknowledged. This enabled the Task Group to make its evaluation on the basis of more complete data.

The efforts of all who helped in the preparation and finalization of the documents are gratefully acknowledged.

* * *

Partial financial support for the publication of this criteria document was kindly provided by the United States Department of Health and Human Services, through a contract from the National Institute of Environmental Health Sciences, Research Triangle Park, North Carolina, USA - a WHO collaborating Centre for Environmental Health Effects. The United Nations Environment Programme (UNEP) generously supported the costs of printing.

* * *

NOTE: The proprietary information contained in this document cannot replace documentation for registration purposes, because the latter has to be closely linked to the source, the manufacturing route, and the purity/impurities of the substance to be registered. The data should be used in accordance with paragraphs 82-84 and recommendations paragraph 90 of the Second FAO Government Consultation (1982).

INTRODUCTION

SYNTHETIC PYRETHROIDS - A PROFILE

1. During investigations to modify the chemical structures of natural pyrethrins, a certain number of synthetic pyrethroids were produced with improved physical and chemical properties and greater biological activity. Several of the earlier synthetic pyrethroids were successfully commercialized, mainly for the control of household insects. Other more recent pyrethroids have been introduced as agricultural insecticides because of their excellent activity against a wide range of insect pests and their non-persistence in the environment.

2. The pyrethroids constitute another group of insecticides in addition to organochlorine, organophosphorus, carbamate, and other compounds. Pyrethroids commercially available to date include allethrin, resmethrin, d-phenothrin, and tetramethrin (for insects of public health importance), and cypermethrin, deltamethrin, fenvalerate, and permethrin (mainly for agricultural insects). Other pyrethroids are also available including furamethrin, kadethrin, and tellallethrin (usually for household insects), fenpropathrin, tralomethrin, cyhalothrin, lambda-cyhalothrin, tefluthrin, cyfluthrin, flucythrinate, fluvalinate, and biphenate (for agricultural insects).

3. Toxicological evaluations of several synthetic pyrethroids have been performed by the FAO/WHO Joint Meeting on Pesticide Residues (JMPR). The acceptable daily intake (ADI) or temporary ADI has been estimated by the JMPR for cypermethrin, deltamethrin, fenvalerate, permethrin, phenothrin, cyfluthrin, cyhalothrin, and flucythrinate.

4. Chemically, synthetic pyrethroids are esters of specific acids (e.g., chrysanthemic acid, halo-substituted chrysanthemic acid, 2-(4-chlorophenyl)-3-methylbutyric acid) and alcohols (e.g., allethrolone, 3-phenoxybenzyl alcohol). For certain pyrethroids, the asymmetric centre(s) exist in the acid and/or alcohol moiety, and the commercial products sometimes consist of a mixture of both optical (1R/1S or d/l) and geometric (cis/trans)-isomers. However, most of the insecticidal activity of such products may reside in only one or two isomers. Some of the products (e.g., d-phenothrin, deltamethrin) consist only of such active isomer(s).

5. Synthetic pyrethroids are neuropoisons acting on the axons in the peripheral and central nervous systems by interacting with sodium channels in mammals and/or insects. A single dose produces toxic signs in mammals, such as tremors, hyperexcitability, salivation, choreoathetosis, and paralysis. The signs disappear fairly rapidly, and the animals recover, generally within a week. At near-lethal dose levels, synthetic pyrethroids cause transient changes in the nervous system, such as axonal swelling and/or breaks and myelin degeneration in sciatic nerves. They are not considered to cause delayed neurotoxicity of the kind induced by some organophosphorus compounds. The mechanism of toxicity of synthetic pyrethroids and their classification into two types are discussed in the Appendix.

6. Some pyrethroids (e.g., deltamethrin, fenvalerate, flucythrinate, and cypermethrin) may cause a transient itching and/or burning sensation in exposed human skin.

7. Synthetic pyrethroids are generally metabolized in mammals through ester hydrolysis, oxidation, and conjugation, and there is no tendency to accumulate in tissues. In the environment, synthetic pyrethroids are fairly rapidly degraded in soil and in plants. Ester hydrolysis and oxidation at various sites on the molecule are the major degradation processes. The pyrethroids are strongly adsorbed on soil and sediments, and hardly eluted with water. There is little tendency for bioaccumulation in organisms.

8. Because of low application rates and rapid degradation in the environment, residues in food are generally low.

9. Synthetic pyrethroids have been shown to be toxic for fish, aquatic arthropods, and honey-bees in laboratory tests. But, in practical usage, no serious adverse effects have been noticed, because of the low rates of application and lack of persistence in the environment. The toxicity of synthetic pyrethroids in birds and domestic animals is low.

10. In addition to the evaluation documents of FAO/WHO, there are several reviews and books on the chemistry, metabolism, mammalian toxicity, environmental effects, etc. of synthetic pyrethroids, including those by Elliot (1977), Miyamoto (1981), Miyamoto & Kearney (1983), and Leahey (1985).

1. SUMMARY

1.1 Identity, Physical and Chemical Properties, Analytical Methods

Resmethrin was first produced in 1967 and marketed in 1969. Chemically, it is an ester of chrysanthemic acid (CA), 2,2-dimethyl-3-(2,2-dimethylvinyl) cyclopropanecarboxylic acid and 5-benzyl-3-furylmethyl alcohol (BFA). It is a racemic mixture of 4 optical isomers: [1R,*trans*]-, [1R,*cis*]-, [1S,*trans*]- and [1S,*cis*]-isomer. The composition ratio in technical products is roughly 4:1:4:1. The [1R,*trans*]-isomer is called bioresmethrin and the [1R,*cis*]-isomer is cismethrin. Among the isomers, the [1R,*trans*]-isomer has the highest insecticidal activity followed by the [1R,*cis*]-isomer.

Technical grade resmethrin is a colourless waxy solid with a melting point of 43-48 °C and a boiling point of 180 °C at 0.01 mmHg. The specific gravity is 1.050 at 20 °C. The vapour pressure is 1.1×10^{-8} mmHg at 30 °C. It is insoluble in water (< 1 mg/litre at 30 °C), but soluble in organic solvents, such as hexane, kerosene, and xylene. It is not stable in air, light, or in alkaline media. The *n*-octanol/water partition coefficient is 2.9×10^3 for resmethrin and 6.2×10^4 for bioresmethrin.

Analysis of environmental samples and determination of residues can be carried out by a high-performance liquid chromatograph equipped with a UV-detector (206 nm) detecting levels as low as 0.05 mg/kg. A gas chromatograph with flame ionization detector is used for the analysis of technical products.

Vapourized resmethrin can be efficiently recovered for analysis by using Porpak C18 or Chromosorb 102 sorbents as the trap.

1.2 Production and Uses

It is estimated that about 20-30 tonnes of resmethrin are produced and used per year. Resmethrin is used mainly for the control of household and public health insects. It is formulated as an aerosol, oil formulation, or emulsifiable concentrate. Formulations are also prepared containing other insecticides and/or synergists.

Bioresmethrin is used on stored grain and for the control of white fly in greenhouses, as well as for household and public health insect control.

1.3 Residues in Food

Resmethrin on treated crops (tomato, lettuce) degraded so that residues were negligible after 3 days on tomato and

< 0.1 mg/kg after 7 days on lettuce. Bioresmethrin on stored grain was fairly stable, a residue of 4 mg/kg declining to 1.1 mg/kg over a period of 6 months. White bread made from treated grain does not contain any residues of resmethrin, but residues may occur in wholemeal bread.

When the cis- and trans-isomers of radiolabelled resmethrin were given orally to White Leghorn laying hens at a dose level of 10 mg/kg, more than 90% of the radioactivity was eliminated in the excreta 24 h after treatment. Residues in the egg white and yolk, and in the body tissues were low, the highest levels occurring in the liver and kidney.

Lactating Jersey cows treated orally with radiolabelled resmethrin at 10 mg/kg body weight rapidly absorbed, metabolized, and excreted the chemical. The cis-isomer was eliminated primarily in the faeces and the trans-isomer was eliminated mainly in the urine. Tissue residues 48 h after treatment were low (< 1 µg/g) except in the liver and kidney, and only very low levels of radioactivity were secreted in the milk.

1.4 Environmental Fate

Resmethrin is rapidly photodegraded on silica gel plates, as a thin film on glass plates, and in aqueous solution. In sunlight, aqueous solutions have a half-life of 47 min (pure water) and 20 min (sea water). A range of photoproducts is formed from ester cleavage and oxidation reactions.

Resmethrin is also very rapidly degraded in soil, 2% of the applied parent compound remaining after 16 days. Complete mineralization to carbon dioxide is a very important degradation process (38% after 16 days).

Rapid degradation occurs on plants (tomato, lettuce, and wheat). After 5 days, no resmethrin is detected on plants and a very complex mixture of, at least, 31 break-down products is formed. The alcohol formed by ester cleavage, benzaldehyde, phenylacetic acid, benzoic acid, and benzyl alcohol were identified as break-down products, each being present at low levels (3% of the total residue).

1.5 Kinetics and Metabolism

When rats were administered ^{14}C-(alcohol labelled)-[1RS, trans]-resmethrin orally at the rate of 500 mg/kg body weight, the radiocarbon was eliminated slowly in the urine (36%) and faeces (64%) within 3 weeks. More than 50% of the ^{14}C dose was secreted in the bile in 72 h and enterohepatically circulated. The major metabolic reactions were ester cleavage, oxidation at the trans-methyl of the isobutenyl group to alcohol, aldehyde, and carboxylic acid and at the

4'-, α-, and 4-positions of 5-benzyl-3-furylmethyl alcohol (BFA), and conjugation.

Rats fed ^{14}C-(acid- or alcohol-labelled) bioresmethrin or cismethrin at the rate of 1 mg/kg eliminated 5-benzyl-3-furancarboxylic acid (BFCA), 4'-hydroxy-BFCA, and α-hydroxy-BFCA together with 2-*trans*- hydroxymethyl- and 2-carboxyl derivatives of chrysanthemic acid (CA). *Cis/trans*-isomerized CA derivatives were also found. The residual metabolites in the body were derived from the alcohol moiety of bioresmethrin.

1.6 Effects on Experimental Animals and In Vitro Test Systems

Resmethrin and bioresmethrin were weakly toxic for animals when examined by various routes of exposure (the oral LD_{50} of resmethrin ranged from 690 mg/kg for the mouse to >5 000 mg/kg for the rat). The oral LD_{50}s for bioresmethrin were 225 mg/kg for the rabbit, 480-10 000 mg/kg for the mouse, and 8800 mg/kg for the rat. Cismethrin was moderately toxic for the mouse (oral LD_{50}: 152-160 mg/kg).

Signs of poisoning were tremors, hyperactivity, and convulsion (T-syndrome). Resmethrin belongs to the Type I pyrethroid group.

The acute toxicity (oral and intraperitoneal) of the metabolites (e.g., CA, BFA, BFCA) was examined in mice and rats; CA and BFA were more toxic than the parent compound in mice though toxic signs were different. The acute toxicity (oral LD_{50}) of the metabolites in rats ranged from 997 mg/kg to > 4640 mg/kg, which is within the same range of acute toxicity as the parent compound. While technical grade resmethrin was found to be a slight irritant to the skin, it did not cause sensitization and photochemical irritation in guinea-pigs and New Zealand White rabbits.

Resmethrin was applied twice weekly, for 3 weeks, to the skin of New Zealand White rabbits by fixing a piece of cotton cloth treated with resmethrin (0.247 mg/cm^2) over skin that had been pre-treated with liquid, imitating sweat, or with resmethrin (10 g), or had not been pre-treated. No significant changes were noted in body weight and organ weight ratios on day 24 or in the clinical chemistry in any of the groups up to day 24. No significant compound-related dermal effects were observed.

When Sprague-Dawley or Long-Evans rats were fed resmethrin in the diet at levels of up to 6000 mg/kg for 14 days, mortality was observed at the highest dose level, and tremor and reduced body weight and food consumption were noted at levels of 1500 mg/kg or more. The maximum no-observed-adverse-effect dietary level was 188 mg/kg for Long-Evans rats.

When Long-Evans rats were given resmethrin in the diet at levels of up to 750 mg/kg (male) and up to 2400 mg/kg (female) for 90 days, all females died at 2400 mg/kg and tremor and reduced body weight were noted at 750 mg/kg. The maximum no-observed-adverse-effect dietary level was 75 mg/kg for both female and male rats.

When rats were fed bioresmethrin in the diet at levels of up to 8000 mg/kg for 91 days, body weight was reduced at the highest level, and was accompanied by changes in blood chemistry indicating liver dysfunction. The no-observed-adverse-effect level in this study was 400 mg/kg diet, which corresponds to 32.8 mg/kg body weight and 36.1 mg/kg body weight for males and females, respectively.

Dogs (males and females) were administered bioresmethrin at levels of up to 500 mg/kg body weight for 90 days. A no-observed-adverse-effect level was observed of 80 mg/kg body weight.

Technical resmethrin was administered via inhalation to Wistar rats for 6 h/day on 5 days of each week, for a period of 90 days, at nominal exposure levels of 0.1, 0.3, or 1.0 g/m^3. The no-observed-adverse-effect level was at 0.1 g/m^3.

Rats and rabbits inhaled aerosolized resmethrin formulations for 5 h/day on 5 consecutive days at levels of 2.9-3.2 mg active ingredient/litre of air. Though clinical signs including rapid breathing and nasal discharge were observed, there were no compound-related effects on body weight and histopathological findings, immediately and 7 and 14 days after exposure. No indication of toxic effects other than irritation were observed in any of the tests.

No oncogenic effects were seen when CD-1 mice were fed 0, 250, 500, or 1000 mg resmethrin/kg basal diet for 85 weeks.

Wistar rats fed resmethrin at levels of 0, 500, 2500, or 5000 mg/kg basal diet for 112 weeks did not show any signs of oncogenicity and a no-observed-adverse-effect level of 500 mg/kg was established for chronic toxicity. When resmethrin was administered to Sprague-Dawley rats at dietary levels of 500, 1500, or 5000 mg/kg for 24 weeks, tremors, decreased body weight, and increased liver and kidney weights were observed at 5000 mg/kg. A no-observed-adverse-effect level of 1500 mg/kg was established.

Dogs fed resmethrin for 6 months showed increased liver weights at 30 mg/kg body weight per day, but did not show any adverse effects at 10 mg/kg body weight per day.

Resmethrin, bioresmethrin, and cismethrin were tested for mutagenicity and/or chromosomal effects in several short-term test systems, such as *Escherichia coli* and *Salmonella* reverse mutation tests, primary DNA damage tests in eukaryotes and prokaryotes, and chromosomal effects in Chinese hamster cells or mouse bone marrow cells. Negative results were obtained with all tests.

In a teratogenicity study, pregnant Long-Evans rats were administered resmethrin in the diet at levels of 188 or 1500 mg/kg, from day 6 to day 16 of gestation. Though mortality, tremor, and decreased food and water consumption were noted in the dams at 1500 mg/kg, gross abnormalities of the fetal skeleton and soft tissues were not observed in the treated animals.

Resmethrin was administered orally (by gavage in corn oil) at levels of 0, 20, 40, or 80 mg/kg body weight to female Sprague-Dawley rats during the period of major organogenesis. Resmethrin was not teratogenic at levels up to and including 80 mg/kg. The no-observed-adverse-effect level for fetotoxicity was 40 mg/kg.

ICR mice were given (+),-[*trans*, *cis*]-resmethrin orally at levels up to 100 mg/kg body weight. Sprague-Dawley rats received levels up to 50 mg/kg body weight during the period of major organogenesis. Embryo- and fetotoxicity and teratogenicity were not observed in this study.

In another study, resmethrin was administered to New Zealand White rabbits by oral intubation at dose levels of 0, 10, 30, or 100 mg/kg body weight on day 6 to day 18 of gestation. Resmethrin was not teratogenic at levels up to and including the 100 mg/kg dose.

In a 3-generation reproduction study, Sprague-Dawley rats were fed resmethrin in the basal diet at 0, 500, 800, or 1250 mg/kg. A decrease in pup weight and a slight increase in the number of pups cast dead were observed at the 500 mg/kg.

1.7 Effects on the Environment

In laboratory studies, resmethrin is highly toxic for fish with 96-h LC_{50} values of 0.3-5.5 µg/litre. Among the isomers, cismethrin is the most toxic for fish. However, under field conditions, it has been shown that the hazard is significantly reduced because of the rapid degradation and low water solubility of the compound. Resmethrin is less toxic for arthropods with 48-h LC_{50} values of 2-25 µg/litre. Both bioresmethrin and cismethrin are harmless for birds.

2. IDENTITY, PHYSICAL AND CHEMICAL PROPERTIES, ANALYTICAL METHODS

2.1 Identity

Chemical formula: $C_{22}H_{26}O_3$

Chemical structure:

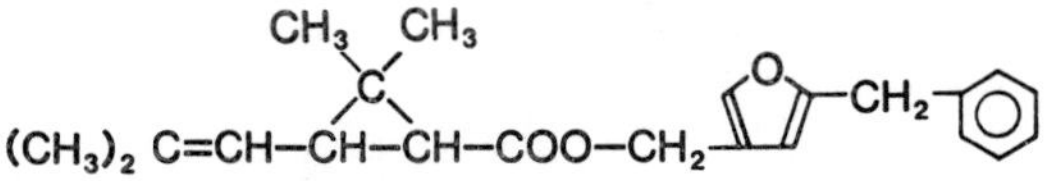

Resmethrin was first produced in 1967 by Elliott et al. (1967). It is prepared by the esterification of [1RS, 3RS or 1RS, <u>cis</u>, <u>trans</u>]-2,2-dimethyl-3-(2,2-dimethylvinyl)cyclopropanecarboxylic acid or chrysanthemic acid with 5-benzyl-3-furylmethyl alcohol.

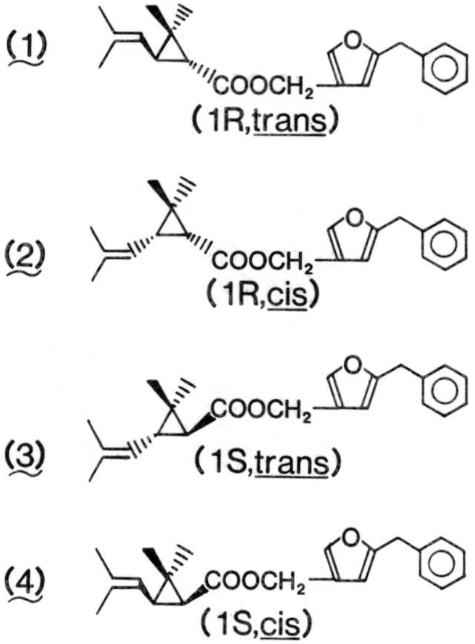

Fig. 1. Chemical structures of 4 stereoisomers.

Resmethrin is thus a mixture of 4 stereoisomers (see Fig. 1). The cis:trans isomer ratio is reported to be 1:4 and the optical ratio of 1R:1S is 1:1 (racemic). Thus, its composition will be roughly 4:1:4:1 of isomers (1), (2), (3), and (4).

Bioresmethrin is the [1R,trans]- or (1) isomer and cismethrin is the [1R,cis]- or (2) isomer (Table 1).

2.2 Physical and Chemical Properties

Some physical and chemical properties of resmethrins are given in Table 2.

Resmethrin is decomposed rapidly on exposure to air or light and in alkaline media (Elliot, 1976; FAO/WHO, 1976; Martin & Worthing, 1977; Meister et al., 1983; Puchalski, 1983; Worthing & Walker, 1983; Devaux & Bolla, 1986).

2.3 Analytical Methods

Methods for the determination of residues, analysis of environmental samples, and product analysis for both resmethrin and bioresmethrin are summarized in Table 3. Procedures for extraction, partition, and cleanup are listed together with analytical equipment and conditions, minimum detectable concentrations, and percentage recovery.

Technical grade resmethrin can be analysed by dissolving the product and dicyclohexyl phthalate (an internal standard) in acetone and injecting the solution in a gas chromatograph equipped with a flame ionization detector (FID) (Murano, 1972).

The sampling efficiency for vapourized pesticides (chlordane, chlorpyrifos, diazinone, propoxur, and resmethrin) was examined using five trapping solid sorbents, i.e., polyurethane foam, dispo plugs, Chromosorb 102, Porpak C18, Carbowax 20M on Gas Chrom Q, and Tenax GC (Roper & Wright, 1984). Resmethrin was determined using HPLC. The sampling efficiency of Porpak C18 was best (94%) for resmethrin; however, that of Chromosorb 102 was best (95%) when means of the 5 sorbents with the different insecticides were compared.

Table 1. Chemical identity of resmethrins of various stereoisomeric compositions

Common name/ CAS Registry No./ RTECS Registry No.[a]	CAS Index name (9CI) Stereospecific name[b,c]	Stereoisomeric composition[d]	Synonyms and trade names
Resmethrin[e] 10453-86-8 GZ1310000	[5-(phenylmethyl)-3-furanyl]methyl 2,2-dimethyl-3-(2-methyl-1-propenyl)cyclopropanecarboxylate (9CI) 5-benzyl-3-furylmethyl [1RS, *cis*, *trans*]-2,2-dimethyl-3-(2,2-dimethylvinyl)-cyclopropanecarboxylate or 5-benzyl-3-furylmethyl [1RS, *cis*, *trans*]-chrysanthemate	(1):(2):(3):(4) =4:1:4:1	Benzofuroline, Benzylfuroline, Chrysron, Chryson, Synthrin, For-Syn, NIA17370, NRDC104, SBP-1382, ENT27474, FMC17370, RU 48440, Pynosect, Pyretherm, Premgard
Bioresmethrin[e] 28434-01-7 GZ1310500	same as resmethrin 5-benzyl-3-furylmethyl [1R, *trans*]-chrysanthemate	(1)	d-*trans*-Resmethrin, (+)-*trans*-Resmethrin, NRDC107, RU 11484,
Cismethrin 35764-59-1 GZ1430000	same as resmethrin 5-benzyl-3-furylmethyl [1R, *cis*]-chrysanthemate	(2)	(+)-*cis*-Resmethrin, NRDC119

Table 1 (contd).

Common name/ CAS Registry No./ RTECS Registry No.[a]	CAS Index name (9CI) Stereospecific name[b,c]	Stereoisomeric composition[d]	Synonyms and trade names
(-)-*trans*-resmethrin	same as resmethrin	(3)	-
GZ1410000	5-benzyl-3-furylmethyl [1S, *trans*]-chrysanthemate		
(-)-*cis*-resmethrin GZ 1420000	same as above	(4)	-
	5-benzyl-3-furylmethyl [1S, *cis*]-chrysanthemate		

[a] NIOSH (1983).
[b] (1R), d, (+) or (1S), 1, (-) in the acid part of resmethrin signifies the same stereospecific conformation, respectively.
[c] Chrysanthemic acid is a name of the acid that forms the acid part of resmethrin.
[d] Numbers in the parentheses identify the structures shown in the figures of stereoisomers.
[e] ISO common name: Common names for pesticides and other agrochemicals approved by the Technical Committee of the International Organization for Standardization.

Table 2. Some physical and chemical properties of resmethrins

	Resmethrin	Bioresmethrin	Cismethrin
Physical state	waxy solid	Viscous oil (liquid or solid)	--
Colour	colourless	practically colourless	--
Relative molecular mass	338.48	338.48	338.48
Melting point (°C)	43 - 48	30 - 35	--
Boiling point	180 °C (0.01 mmHg)	180 °C (0.01 mmHg)	--
Water solubility (30 °C)	< 1 mg/litre	< 0.3 mg/litre	--
Solubility in organic solvents	soluble[a]	soluble	soluble
Density (20 °C)	1.050	1.050	
Vapour pressure (mmHg)	1.1×10^{-8} (30 °C)	1.4×10^{-4} (25 °C)	--
n-Octanol/water partition coefficient	2.9×10^{3}	6.2×10^{4}	

[a] Methanol (81 g/kg), hexane (220 g/kg), xylene (> 1kg/kg), kerosene (10%). Very soluble in methylene chloride and aromatic petroleum hydrocarbons.

Table 3. Analytical methods for resmethrin[a]

Sample	Sample preparation				Determination	Limit of detection (mg/kg)	% Recovery (fortification level mg/kg)	Reference
	Extraction solvent	Partition	Clean-up		GC or HPLC condition, detector, carrier, flow, column, temperature, R.T.			
			Column	Elution				
Residue analysis								
Apple Pear Cabbage Potato	n-hexane/ acetone (1/1)	extraction solvent/ H_2O	silica gel	CH_2Cl_2	HPLC UV-206 nm, 25 cm ODS, propane 2-ol, 1 ml/min	0.05 0.05 0.05 0.05	37 (0.1), 60 (1.0) 44 (0.1), 72 (1.0) 34 (0.1), 57 (1.0) 54 (0.1), 80 (1.0)	Baker & Bottomley (1982)
Corn Cornmeal Flour Wheat	pentane	CH_3CN/ pentane	Florisil	EtOAc/ pentane (3 + 97)	FID-GC, N_2 86 ml/min, 1.83 m, 10% UC-W 98, 245 °C, 5.5 min	0.2	80 - 87.5 (0.2 - 3.2) 75 - 86.2 (0.15 - 2.56) 80 - 88.7 (0.16 - 2.71) 79.6 - 86.2 (0.16 - 2.55)	Simonaitis & Cail (1975)
Wheat (grain)	n-hexane				CI-MS/GC, m/e 171, methane, 20 ml/min, 1.5 m, 5% OV-101, 230 °C, ca. 2.5 min	0.04	97 (0.2) 98 (1.0) 92 (2.0)	Cave (1981)
Rice (cooked)	petroleum ether acetone acetone/ petroleum ether (2/8)				colorimetric method, 680 nm		96 (0.7) 93 (0.8) 93 (0.8)	Desmarchelier (1980)

Table 3 (contd).

Sample	Sample preparation				Determination	Limit of detection (mg/kg)	% Recovery (fortification level mg/kg)	Reference
	Extraction solvent	Partition	Clean-up		GC or HPLC condition, detector, carrier, flow, column, temperature, R.T.			
			Column	Elution				
Environmental analysis								
Dish Apple Spinach (dislodgeable residue)	n-hexane	n-hexane/ CH_3CN	HPTLC	benzene/ CCl_4 (1 + 1) Rf = 0.44	dual-wavelength densitometry λ1 = 370 nm; λ2 = 230 nm		88 - 98 (300 µg) 97 (300 µg) 98 (300 µg)	Uno et al. (1982)
Product analysis								
Technial grade	acetone				FID-GC, H_2 40 ml/min, 1 m, 2% DEGS, 190 °C, 3.9 min			Murano (1972)

a HPLC = high-performance liquid chromatography; FID = Flame ionization detector; MS = mass spectrometry; CC = column chromatography; GC = gas chromatography; UV = ultraviolet; HPTLC = high-performance thin-layer chromatography; RT = retention time; CI = chemical ionization.

3. SOURCES OF ENVIRONMENTAL POLLUTION AND ENVIRONMENTAL LEVELS

3.1 Industrial Production

Resmethrin was first put on the market in 1969 and bioresmethrin, in 1973. No information is available to the general public on production volume. However, it has been estimated to amount to 20-30 tonnes yearly (Miyamoto, personal communication, 1986).

3.2 Use Patterns

Resmethrin is mainly used in aerosol formulations, but also in oil formulations and emulsifiable concentrates, for the control of household and public health insects. It is also used in combination with other insecticides (e.g., tetramethrin, malathion).

Resmethrin is currently used for mosquito control (by aerial application) in the USA, and it can also be used for the control of white fly in greenhouses.

Bioresmethrin is mainly used as a post-harvest treatment to control pests in stored grain (mostly in Australia). Bioresmethrin is also widely used for white fly control in greenhouse-grown vegetables, mostly in European countries. It is also used in aerosol formulation for the control of household and public health insects, in combination with synergists and/or other insecticides. It has been used in France for cattle shed treatment (Battelle, 1982).

3.3 Residues in Food

Resmethrin residues on tomatoes and lettuce after greenhouse treatment decreased very rapidly resulting in negligible residues on tomatoes after 3 days and < 0.1 mg/kg on lettuce after 7 days (Burt, 1983a,b).

Field trials have been carried out with bioresmethrin on fruit and vegetable crops, e.g., tomatoes and cucumbers. Tomato fruits were treated with ^{14}C-labelled bioresmethrin (1.25 mg/kg). The fruit was harvested 7-72 h after application and amounts of the compound in the flesh and skin, and on the skin surface were measured. At 72 h, 0.2% of the applied compound was detected in the flesh, 4.65% in the skin, and 15.5% on the surface (Buick & Flanagan, 1973).

There are many reports of residue studies, especially on post-harvest treatment of grain for storage (FAO/WHO, 1976/1977).

Residues in the stored grains, e.g., wheat, have also been determined. For example, wheat was treated with bioresmethrin at the rate of 4 mg/kg and maintained in an unaerated silo at 24 °C or in an aerated silo at 14 °C, for 6 months. At the end of 6 months, the residue levels had declined to only 1.1 mg/kg (unaerated) and 1.9 mg/kg (aerated) (Bengston et al., 1975).

Wheat was treated with bioresmethrin (4 mg/kg) and subjected to milling and baking processes. When it was used with 20 mg piperonyl butoxide/kg, 4.0 mg bioresmethrin remained per kg flour, but no residues were detected in bread (Ardley, 1975). In another study, some stability of residues during baking were demonstrated, residues of 2.9 mg/kg in wheat resulted in residues of 1 mg/kg in wholemeal bread (Desmarchelier, 1980).

3.4 Fate and Residues in Domestic Animals

White Leghorn laying hens were given the *cis*- and *trans*-isomers of resmethrin, labelled with radiocarbon in either the alcohol or acid moiety, at a dosage of 10 mg/kg body weight. With each isomer and label position, more than 90% of the radiocarbon was eliminated in the excreta within 24 h of the treatment. Radiocarbon residues in the egg white and yolk fractions were low with peak levels observed, respectively, 1 and 4-5 days after treatment. Radiocarbon residues in tissues were low in birds sacrificed 12 h after treatment. The highest levels were found in the liver and kidney (Christopher et al., 1985).

Resmethrin labelled with radiocarbon in either the acid or alcohol moiety and administered orally to lactating Jersey cows at 10 mg/kg body weight was rapidly absorbed, metabolized, and excreted. The *cis*-isomer was eliminated primarily in the faeces, but the *trans*-isomer was eliminated primarily in the urine. Tissue residues 48 h after treatment were low (< 1 mg/kg), except in the liver, ovary, and kidney, and were generally higher with the alcohol-labelled compounds. Only very low levels of radiocarbon were secreted in the milk. Unmetabolized resmethrin appeared in trace amounts in tissues and as the major residue in milk and faeces. The major metabolites from both isomers arise from ester hydrolysis and subsequent oxidation of the hydrolysed products. They include: chrysanthemic acid (free and conjugated with glucuronic acid), chrysanthemumdicarboxylic acid, 5-benzyl-3-furoic acid (free and conjugated with glucuronic acid or glycine), and 5-(α-hydroxybenzyl)-3-furoic acid (Ridlen et al., 1984).

4. ENVIRONMENTAL TRANSPORT, DISTRIBUTION AND TRANSFORMATION

4.1 Photodegradation

The photodegradation pathways of resmethrin are summarized in Fig. 2.

On irradiation with a sunlamp, trans- and cis-isomers of ^{14}C-resmethrin (5) labelled in the carboxy (acid) or phenyl (alcohol) group decomposed on silica gel plates with a half-life of about 160-190 min. After 420 min irradiation of ^{14}C-bioresmethrin, only 5% of the recovered radioactivity was resmethrin, 45% was ester photoproducts, 14% was non-ester photoproducts, and 32% was not identified. The photoproduct found in the largest amount was 5-hydroxy-3-oxo-4-phenyl-1-cyclopentenylmethyl trans-chrysanthemate (10) (about 24% of the applied ^{14}C), which originated from the cyclic ozonide-type peroxide intermediates (8,9) formed by oxidation of the furan ring. A relatively large (about 5%) amount of trans-chrysanthemic acid (17) was formed. In addition, small amounts of the R and S isomers of trans-epoxyresmethrin (6) (about 1.5% each), 5-benzyl-5-hydroxy-2-oxo-2,5-dihydro-3-furylmethyl trans-chrysanthemate (11) (about 3%) and 2-benzyloxy-5-oxo-2,5-dihydro-3-furylmethyl trans-chrysanthemate (12) (about 1%) were detected with the acid- and alcohol-labelled preparations, and benzyl alcohol (14) (about 2%), benzoic acid (16) (about 1.5%), and phenylacetic acid (13) (about 1%) were found with the alcohol-labelled preparation. The photoproduct distribution was greatly dependent on the supporting material or medium. Oxidation at the furan ring occurred predominantly on silica gel plates, while epoxidation at the isobutenyl substituent proceeded to a greater extent on a filter paper or in water. When exposed to sunlight for 10 h, cismethrin on silica gel plates (1.7 mg/cm^2) gave a large amount of cis-chrysanthemic acid (17) but not trans-acid, together with smaller amounts of 5-hydroxy-3-oxo-4-phenyl-1-cyclopentenylmethyl cis-chrysanthemate (10), 5-benzyl-5-hydroxy-2-oxo-2,5-dihydro-3-furylmethyl cis-chrysanthemate (11), benzaldehyde (15), and phenylacetic acid (13). The photodecomposition rates were compared for residual deposits (14 μg/cm^2) of bio-resmethrin, trans-tetramethrin, and S-Bioallethrin on silica gel plates under sunlight or a sunlamp. S-Bioallethrin was the most stable of these compounds, and trans-tetramethrin was more persistent than bioresmethrin (Ueda et al., 1974).

Resmethrin and structurally related 5-benzyl-3-furylmethyl derivatives undergo rapid oxidation when exposed to sunlight or a sunlamp, either in aqueous medium or as a thin film on

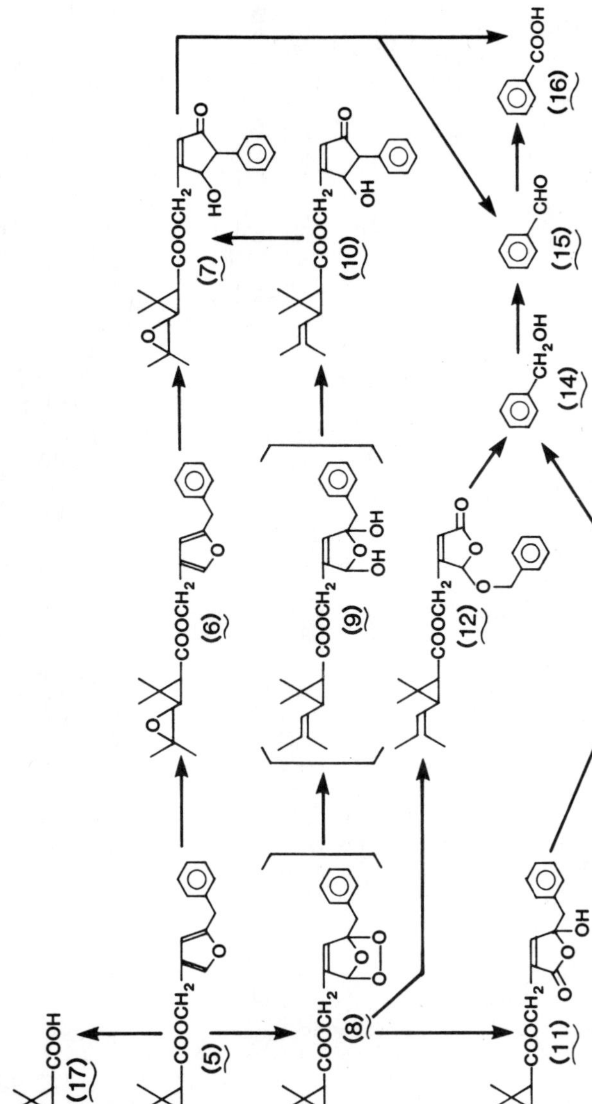

Fig. 2. Photodegradation pathways of resmethrin.

glass or silica gel. One major photodecomposition route involves epoxidation at the isobutenyl substituent to give the R- and S-epoxides. Formation of the other major photoproducts is initiated by oxidation of the furan ring to a cyclic ozonide-type peroxide (Holmstead et al., 1977).

In contrast, there was a 10% loss in the original weight of resmethrin after 24 h compared with losses of 29% and 41% for tetramethrin and allethrin, respectively, when exposed as a thin film (500 mg/38.5 cm^2) on glass to an incandescent lamp (Abe et al., 1972).

The photodegradation of aqueous solutions (sterile water and artificial sea-water) of resmethrin by natural sunlight has also been investigated. The half-life was estimated to be 47 min in water and 20 min in sea water. The major degradation product was chrysanthemic acid (Watson, 1984).

4.2 Degradation in Soil

The degradation under aerobic conditions of ^{14}C-resmethrin applied to soil at rates equivalent to 0.12 and 1.7 kg/ha has been studied. The compound degraded very rapidly, so that less than 2% of the applied ^{14}C-resmethrin remained after 16 days. Complete mineralisation to $^{14}CO_2$ was a very important metabolic process (38% of the applied radioactivity in 16 days). The radioactivity remaining in the soil after 16 days was a complex mixture of more than 11 products resulting from ester cleavage and oxidation reactions (Kaufman, 1986).

4.3 Degradation on Plants

Tomato and lettuce plants were treated with ^{14}C-resmethrin, under greenhouse conditions; wheat was similarly treated in the field. The radioactivity was applied by spraying an aqueous suspension at a concentration equivalent to 0.5 g/litre. The applied resmethrin degraded very rapidly so that 55-82% had degraded within 2 h and no unchanged resmethrin remained after 5 days. A very complex mixture of degradation products were formed on the plants (up to 31 individual compounds). No individual component in the mixture of products formed exceeded 10% of the amount applied at any sampling interval up to 15 days after treatment. The alcohol formed by ester cleavage and benzaldehyde (15), phenylacetic acid (13), benzoic acid (16), and benzyl alcohol (14) were identified as degradation products. These compounds were each present at levels $< 3\%$ of the radioactive residue (Mumma, 1985).

5. KINETICS AND METABOLISM

5.1 Metabolism in Mammals

Metabolic pathways for resmethrin in mammals are summarized in Fig. 3.

When ^{14}C-[1RS,trans]-resmethrin (19) labelled in the alcohol moiety was administered orally to Sprague-Dawley rats at 500 mg/kg, the radiocarbon was rapidly absorbed from the gastrointestinal tract and it took 3 weeks for the complete elimination of the radioactivity in the urine (36% of the dose) and faeces (64%). A negligible amount (less than 0.1%) of the radiocarbon was expired as $^{14}CO_2$. The radiocarbon was not completely excreted, even after 2 weeks, in rats given an intravenous dose of 50 mg/kg; notably, appreciable amounts of ^{14}C were found in faeces. The results of another study indicated that the excretion of ^{14}C via the bile duct was very rapid and that more than 50% of the total dose was recovered from the bile within 72 h. The urinary metabolites were mainly 5-benzyl-3-furancarboxylic acid (20) (BFCA) in the free form (28% of the urinary ^{14}C), the glucuronide form (2%), and unknown conjugated (18%) forms. Other significant metabolites present in the urine were hydroxy derivatives of BFCA, such as α-(4-carboxy-2-furyl)-benzyl alcohol (21) (α-OH-BFCA) (11%), 5-benzoyl-3-furancarboxylic acid (22) (α-keto-BFCA) (1%), 5-benzyl-4-hydroxy-3-furancarboxylic acid (23) (2%), and 5-(p-hydroxybenzyl)-3-furancarboxylic acid (24) (4'-OH-BFCA) in the free form (3%), the sulfate form (12%) and the glucuronide (2%) form (Miyamoto et al., 1971) (Fig. 3).

Ueda et al. (1975b) elucidated the metabolic fates of the acid and alcohol moieties of bioresmethrin (19) and cismethrin (25) in rats after a single oral dose (acid- and alcohol-labelled moieties) at 1 mg/kg. The predominant metabolites from the alcohol moiety were BFCA, 4'-OH-BFCA, and α-OH-BFCA. The metabolites in the body were derived from the alcohol moiety of bioresmethrin. On the other hand, the isobutenyl group of the acid moiety was oxidized at either the cis- or trans-methyl group of cismethrin, but only at the trans-methyl group of bioresmethrin. The major metabolites from the acid moiety were the hydroxymethyl (28,29) or dicarboxylic acid derivatives (30,31) of chrysanthemic acid (26,27) (CA). The aldehyde intermediates of CA were not found. The major dicarboxylic acid derivatives of CA were metabolites receiving oxidation at the trans-methyl group of the isobutenyl moiety. Although the trans-methyl group was predominantly oxidized in both isomers, the cis-methyl group of the cis-isomer was also oxidized(32). An anticipated meta-

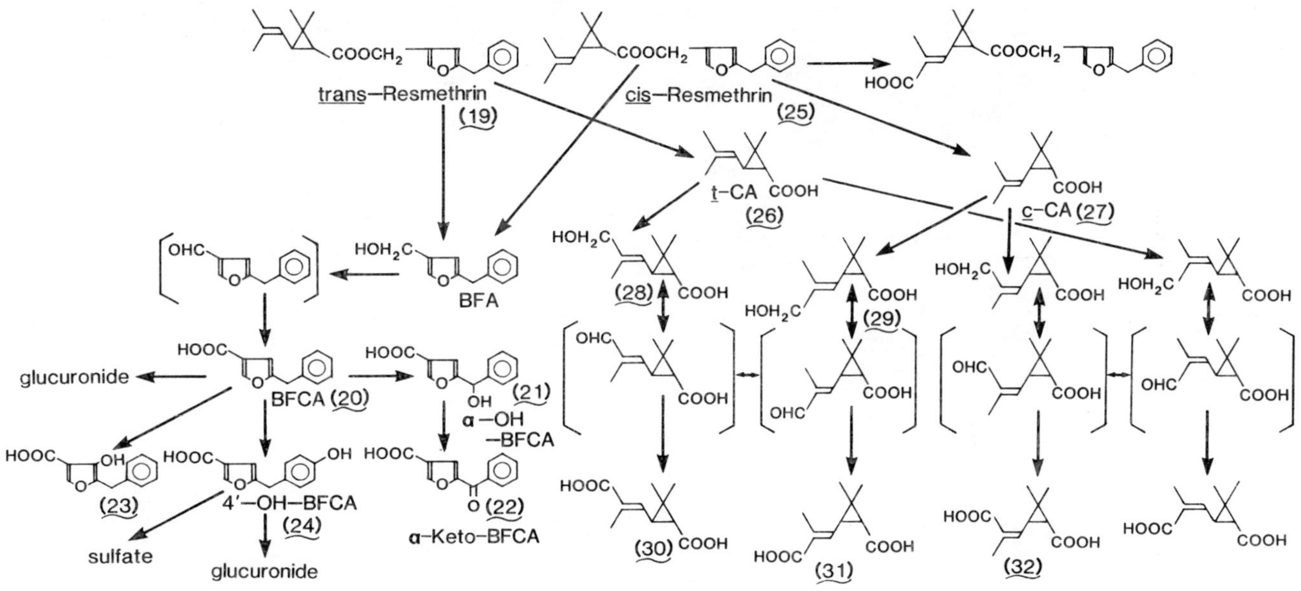

Fig. 3. Metabolic pathways of resmethrin in mammals.

bolic pathway involves epimerization at C-3 of the cyclopropane group leading to isomerized forms of dicarboxylic acid derivatives of CA. The aldehyde derivatives of CA are the most likely compounds for isomerization, because these derivatives readily undergo *cis*- *trans*-isomerization under the alkaline conditions (Ueda et al., 1975b).

5.2 Enzymatic Systems for Biotransformation

When ^{14}C alcohol-labelled cismethrin, bioresmethrin, and 5-benzyl-3-furylmethyl alcohol (BFA) (18) were incubated with rat liver S-9 homogenates or microsomes, a proportion of the radioactive compounds was covalently bound to proteins. The covalent binding was greater with phenobarbital-pretreated rats, and dependent on a NADPH-generating system. When a S-9 homogenate was used, the bound compounds were twice as high for cismethrin as for bioresmethrin and BFA. Inversely, when microsomes were used, more covalent binding occurred with bioresmethrin and BFA than with cismethrin. The inhibition of esterases by tetraethyl pyrophosphate (TEPP) in a S-9 homogenate did not alter the amount of covalent binding to the three compounds, whereas malathion inhibited this binding. However, treatment of a S-9 homogenate with piperonyl butoxide greatly reduced covalent binding. Covalent binding was inhibited when the microsomes were incubated with carbon monoxide or modified by thermal denaturation. It is suggested that oxidative metabolism was responsible for the covalent binding (Hoellinger et al., 1985).

When four resmethrin isomers ([1R,*trans*]-, [1S,*trans*]-, [1R,*cis*]-, and [1S,*cis*]-) were incubated with mouse and rat microsomes in 50 mmol/litre tris-HCl buffer (pH 7.4) at 37 °C for 1 h, microsomal esterases readily cleaved the *trans*- but not the *cis*-isomers. The ester linkage also appeared to undergo oxidative cleavage when esterase attack was minimal. Ester metabolites were detected in significant amounts only with [1R,*cis*]-resmethrin, in which case oxidation had occurred at the isobutenyl moiety, with or without oxidation at the benzylfuryl methyl group. Most of the *in vitro* metabolites were identical with those in the excreta of rats given resmethrin orally. The preferred site of oxidation in the isobutenyl moiety varies with the resmethrin isomer and microsomal source. Mouse microsomes predominantly oxidized the *trans*-methyl group of both [1R,*trans*]- and [1S,*trans*]-resmethrin, the selectivity, however, being the greatest with [1S,*trans*]-resmethrin. Rat microsomes were relatively nonselective in attacking the isobutenyl methyl groups of [1R,*trans*]-resmethrin (Ueda et al., 1975a).

Plasma-esterases were equally active in hydrolysing cismethrin and bioresmethrin(3.2-3.4 nmol benzylfurylmethanol/min per g) whereas liver microsomal esterases hydrolysed bio-resmethrin 10 times more rapidly than cismethrin (White et al., 1976).

6. EFFECTS ON THE ENVIRONMENT

Data on the acute toxicity of resmethrin for aquatic and terrestrial non-target organisms are summarized in Tables 4 and 5, respectively.

6.1 Aquatic Organisms

Resmethrin is highly toxic for fish, and the toxicity is negatively correlated with temperature (Mauck et al., 1976): the LC_{50} value for bluegill is 2.3 times greater at 22 °C than at 12 °C, as shown in Table 4. The influence of both water hardness and pH on toxicity ranged from slight to negligible. By keeping resmethrin solution at 12 °C for 1 week, the toxicity for bluegill decreased 2-fold at each pH value as the resmethrin solution aged.

Among the 4 isomers, the 1R, *cis*-isomer is most toxic for fish, followed by the 1R, *trans*-, 1S, *cis*- and 1S, *trans*-, as observed in pyrethroids. Contrary to other pyrethroids, resmethrin is less toxic for arthropods than for fish, as shown in Table 4. The 48-h LC_{50} values for arthropods are in the range of 2-25 µg/litre (Nishiuchi, 1981).

Laboratory studies have shown that resmethrin is highly toxic for fish but, because of the low water solubility of the compound and rapid environmental degradation (photochemical and microbial), it would be expected that, under field conditions, the toxic impact would be greatly reduced. Such a reduction in toxic effects has been confirmed in field studies carried out in the USA (Sjogren, 1985; Norwood, 1986; Pierce, 1986).

In one of these studies, ponds were sprayed with resmethrin formulations at the expected field rate for adult mosquito control (0.01 kg/ha). Residue analysis confirmed that resmethrin levels fall rapidly (1.1 ppb at zero time non-detectable after 96 h). Caged fish showed good survival (82-100% for bluegill, 73-100% for goldfish) in resmethrin-treated ponds. However, one fish species in this study (white sucker) was susceptible (8% survival) when piperonyl butoxide-synergised resmethrin was used, though good survival was noted for this species with unsynergised resmethrin. In a second study, synergised resmethrin was applied to a mangrove-fringed pond at 2-day intervals. The first two applications were at the normal field rate, but the third was at 10 times this rate. In this study, both fish species used to monitor fish survival (sheepshead minnow, fingerling snook) showed good survival (100% at the normal rate and 88% at the 10-fold rate).

Table 4. Acute toxicity of resmethrin for non-target aquatic organisms

Species	Size	Parameter	Concentration (µg/litre)	Formulation	System	Temperature (°C)	pH	Hardness (mg $CaCO_3$/litre)	Reference
Fish									
Carp (*Cyprinus carpio*)		48-h LC_{50}	44	technical	static	25			Nishiuchi (1982)
Killifish (*Oryzias latipes*)	adult	48-h LC_{50}	300	technical	static	25			Miyamoto (1976)
	adult	48-h LC_{50}	16	(+)-*trans*-	static	25			Miyamoto (1976)
	adult	48-h LC_{50}	8	(+)-*cis*-	static	25			Miyamoto (1976)
	adult	48-h LC_{50}	> 10 000	(-)-*trans*-	static	25			Miyamoto (1976)
	adult	48-h LC_{50}	3500	(-)-*cis*-	static	25			Miyamoto (1976)
Rainbow trout (*Salmo gairdneri*)		96-h LC_{50}	2.2	technical	static	12			Marking & Mauck (1975)
Coho salmon (*Oncorhynchus kisutch*)		96-h LC_{50}	1.50	technical	static	12			Mauck et al. (1976)
		96-h LC_{50}	0.277	technical	flow-through	12			Mauck et al. (1976)
Steelhead trout (*Salmo gairdneri*)		96-h LC_{50}	0.450	technical	static	12			Mauck et al. (1976)
		96-h LC_{50}	0.275	technical	flow-through	12			Mauck et al. (1976)
Yellow perch (*Perca flavescens*)		96-h LC_{50}	2.36	technical	static	12			Mauck et al. (1976)
		96-h LC_{50}	0.513	technical	flow-through	12			Mauck et al. (1976)

Table 4 (contd).

Species	Size	Parameter	Concentration (µg/litre)	Formulation	System	Temperature (°C)	pH	Hardness (mg $CaCO_3$/litre)	Reference
Arthropods									
Daphnia pulex		3-h LC_{50}	15 000	technical	static	25			Nishiuchi (1982)
		3-h LC_{50}	50 000	technical	static	25			Miyamoto (1976)
		3-h LC_{50}	25 000 - 50 000	(+)-trans-	static	25			Miyamoto (1976)
		3-h LC_{50}	25 000 - 50 000	(+)-cis-	static	25			Miyamoto (1976)
		3-h LC_{50}	> 50 000	(-)-trans-	static	25			Miyamoto (1976)
		3-h LC_{50}	> 50 000	(-)-cis-	static	25			Miyamoto (1976)
Moina macrocopa		3-h LC_{50}	14 000	technical	static	25			Nishiuchi (1982)
Sigara substriata	0.59 cm; 6.1 mg	48-h LC_{50}	2	technical	static	25			Nishiuchi (1981)
Micronecta sedula	0.32 cm; 1.8 mg	48-h LC_{50}	3.3	technical	static	25			Nishiuchi (1981)
Cloeon dipterum	0.93 cm; 5.6 mg	48-h LC_{50}	4.5	technical	static	25			Nishiuchi (1981)
Orthetrum albistylum speciosum	2.3 cm; 0.62 g	48-h LC_{50}	7.3	technical	static	25			Nishiuchi (1981)
Eretes sticticus	1.5 cm; 0.2 g	48-h LC_{50}	25	technical	static	25			Nishiuchi (1981)
Sympetrum frequens	2.1 cm; 0.56 g	48-h LC_{50}	10	technical	static	25			Nishiuchi (1981)

Table 4 (contd).

<u>Fish</u> (contd).									
Bluegill (*Lepomis macrochirus*)		96-h LC_{50}	2.62	technical	static	12			Mauck et al. (1976)
		96-h LC_{50}	0.750	technical	flow-through	12			Mauck et al. (1976)
	0.8 g	96-h LC_{50}	5.46	technical	static	22	7.5	40 - 48	Mauck et al. (1976)
	0.8 g	96-h LC_{50}	4.28	technical	static	17	7.5	40 - 48	Mauck et al. (1976)
	0.8 g	96-h LC_{50}	2.33	technical	static	12	7.5	40 - 48	Mauck et al. (1976)
	0.8 g	96-h LC_{50}	2.53	technical	static	12	6.6	10 - 13	Mauck et al. (1976)
	0.8 g	96-h LC_{50}	2.54	technical	static	12	7.8	160 - 180	Mauck et al. (1976)
	0.8 g	96-h LC_{50}	2.06	technical	static	12	8.2	280 - 320	Mauck et al. (1976)
	0.8 g	96-h LC_{50}	2.29	technical	static	12	6.5	40 - 48	Mauck et al. (1976)
	0.8 g	96-h LC_{50}	2.46	technical	static	12	9.5	40 - 48	Mauck et al. (1976)
	0.8 g	96-h LC_{50}	2.89	technical	static	12	6.5	40 - 48	Mauck et al. (1976)
	0.8 g	96-h LC_{50}	2.70	technical	static	12	7.5	40 - 48	Mauck et al. (1976)
	0.8 g	96-h LC_{50}	3.13	technical	static	12	8.5	40 - 48	Mauck et al. (1976)
	0.8 g	96-h LC_{50}	2.68	technical	static	12	9.5	40 - 48	Mauck et al. (1976)

6.2 Terrestrial Organisms

Acute toxicity data show that both resmethrin and bioresmethrin (Table 5) are harmless for birds, as are other pyrethroids.

In addition, a study has been carried out to assess the effects of resmethrin on reproduction in the Mallard duck and Bobwhite quail. The birds were given 12, 60, or 300 mg resmethrin/kg diet for 22 weeks. No effects on reproduction were seen in either species at these dose levels (Roberts et al., 1985a,b).

Table 5. Acute toxicity of resmethrin and bioresmethrin for non-target terrestrial organisms

Species	Compound	Size (days)	Application	Toxicity (mg/kg)	Reference
Bird					
Quail (*Coturnix coturnix japonica*)	Resmethrin	14	diet	LC_{50} > 5000	Hill et al. (1975)
Mallard (*Anas platyrhynchos*)		10	diet	LC_{50} > 5000	Hill et al. (1975)
Chicken	Bioresmethrin		oral	LD_{50} > 10 000	Chesher & Malone (1970a) Wallwork et al. (1970)

7. EFFECTS ON EXPERIMENTAL ANIMALS AND IN VITRO TEST SYSTEMS

7.1 Acute Toxicity

Acute toxic signs produced in experimental animals by exposure to resmethrins include tremor, hyperexcitability, convulsive twitching, prostration, and coma.

LD_{50} data on resmethrin isomers administered orally and by other exposure routes are summarized in Tables 6 and 7, respectively.

These data show that resmethrins are weakly toxic, except for cismethrin, the acute oral toxicity of which is moderate in the mouse.

The results of acute toxicity tests of the resmethrin metabolites are given in Table 8.

Acute (1 h) inhalation studies were performed with 3 aerosol formulations of resmethrin and 2 blank formulations. Groups of 20 male rats and 4 male rabbits inhaled the active ingredient at concentration levels of 12-13.7 mg/litre (value based on the weight loss from each spray can). In addition, 10 exposed and 10 control rats were tested for conditioned avoidance performance immediately following exposure. Laboured breathing was seen generally in the animals. Several rabbits died in both the resmethrin-treated and the blank-formulation groups. In the rats, there were no effects on body weight, or gross or histopathological lesions. However, the conditioned avoidance latency in the resmethrin-treated rats was significantly greater than that in the unexposed controls (Macko et al., 1979).

7.2 Short-term Exposure

7.2.1 Oral administration

Groups of 6 Sprague-Dawley rats from each sex were administered resmethrin in the diet at concentrations of 0, 310-323, 630-660, 1230-1250, 1423-2670, or 1680-5100 mg/kg, for 14 days. Five out of 6 rats died at the highest exposure level in both sexes. Tremor was observed and body weight gain and food utilization were reduced at levels of 1230-1250 mg/kg or more. A significant increase in the hepatic organ-to-body weight ratios was noted in all groups of females and in groups of males fed 630-660 mg/kg or more. Compound-related histopathological changes were not observed in any of the tissues and organs examined. The maximum no-observed-adverse-effect dietary level was 310 mg/kg for male rats only (Swentzel et al., 1977).

Table 6. Acute oral toxicity of resmethrin isomers

Compound	Animal	Sex	LD_{50} (mg/kg body weight)	Reference
Resmethrin	rat	M	> 5000	Miyamoto (1976)
	rat	F	> 5000	Miyamoto (1976)
	rat	M	1244	Gaines & Linder (1986)
	rat	F	1721	Gaines & Linder (1986)
	rat (weanling)	M	1987	Gaines & Linder (1986)
	rat	?	> 2500	Worthing & Walker (1983)
	rat	-	960	Volkov et al. (1979)
	mouse	M	690	Miyamoto (1976)
	mouse	F	940	Miyamoto (1976)
Bioresmethrin	rat	M	8800	Glomot & Chevalier (1969)
	rat	F	> 8000	Verschoyle & Barnes (1972)
	rat	F	7071	Wallwork et al. (1970)
	rat	-	840	Kholmatova, (1984)
	rat	-	990	Volkov et al. (1979)
	rat	-	675	Kagan et al. (1986)
	mouse	M	590	Miyamoto (1976)
	mouse	F	800	Miyamoto (1976)
	mouse	M	3100	Ueda et al. (1975b)
	mouse	F	10000	Wallwork et al. (1970)
	mouse	-	520	Kholmatova (1984)
	mouse	-	480	Kagan et al. (1986)
	rabbit	-	225	Kholmatova (1984)
Cismethrin	mouse	M	152	Miyamoto (1976)
	mouse	F	160	Miyamoto (1976)
[1S,-_trans_]-resmethrin	mouse	M	500	Miyamoto (1976)
	mouse	F	600	Miyamoto (1976)
[1S,-_cis_]-resmethrin	mouse	M	3700	Miyamoto (1976)
	mouse	F	5000	Miyamoto (1976)

Table 7. Acute toxicity of resmethrins via other than oral exposure

Compound	Animal	Sex	Route	LD_{50} (mg/kg body weight)	LC_{50} (mg/m^3)	Reference
Resmethrin	rat	M	dermal	2500		Gaines & Linder (1986)
	rat	F	dermal	2500		Gaines & Linder (1986)
	rabbit	-	dermal	2500		Green (1977)
	rat	-	inhalation (4-h exposure)		> 9490	Jackson & Hardy (1984)
	rat	-	inhalation (1-h exposure)		> 12 000	Macko et al. (1979)
	rabbit	-	inhalation (1-h exposure)		> 12 000	Macko et al. (1979)
	dog	-	inhalation (4-h exposure)		> 420	Macko et al. (1979)
Bioresmethrin	rat	F	dermal	> 10 000		Wallwork et al. (1970)
	rat	F	intravenous	340		Verschoyle & Barnes (1972)
	rat	F	intravenous	106-133		Chesher & Malone (1971b)
	rat	F	intraperitoneal	> 8000		Wallwork & Malone (1971)
	rat	F	inhalation (24-h exposure)		> 872	Wallwork & Malone (1972)
	mouse	M	intraperitoneal	> 1500		Ueda et al. (1975b)
	mouse	F	intraperitoneal	> 5359		Wallwork et al. (1970)
Mixture of bioresmethrin & cismethrin	rat	M,F	inhalation (4-h exposure)		> 1500	Miyamoto (1976)
	mouse	M,F	inhalation (4-h exposure)		> 1500	Miyamoto (1976)

Table 8. Acute toxicity of metabolites of resmethrin

Metabolite	No[b]	Animal	LD_{50} (mg/kg) ip	LD_{50} (mg/kg) oral	Reference
(bioresmethrin), (5-benzyl-3-furylmethyl (+)-*trans*-chrysanthemate)	(1)	mouse	> 1500[a]	3100[a]	Miyamoto (1975-1976) Ueda et al. (1975b)
1R or (+)-*cis*-resmethrin (5-benzyl-3-furylmethyl (+)-*cis*-chrysanthemate)	(2)	mouse	320[a]		Miyamoto (1975-1976) Ueda et al. (1975b)
d,l-*cis*,*trans*-chrysanthemic acid	(17)	rat		2443	Reagan & Becci (1985a)
d,l-*trans*-chrysanthemic acid	-	rat		1598	Reagan & Becci (1985b)
(+)-*trans*-chrysanthemic acid, (+)-*trans*-CA (*t*-CA)	(26)	mouse	98[a]	280[a]	Miyamoto (1975-1976) Ueda et al. (1975b)
(+)-*cis*-chrysanthemic acid, (+)-*cis*-CA (*c*-CA)	(27)	mouse	600[a]		Miyamoto (1975-1976) Ueda et al. (1975b)
d-*trans*-chrysanthemic acid	(26)	rat		983	Reagan & Becci (1985c)
(+)-*trans*-chrysanthemumdicarboxylic acid, (+)-*trans*-CDA (*t*E-CDA)	(30)	mouse	408[a]		Miyamoto (1975-1976) Ueda et al. (1975b)
5-benzyl-3-furylmethanol (BFA)	(18)	mouse	75[a]	310[a]	Miyamoto (1975-1976) Ueda et al. (1975b)
5-benzyl-3-furoic acid (BFCA)	(20)	mouse	46[a]		Miyamoto (1975-1976) Ueda et al. (1975b)
5-benzyl-3-furoic acid (BFCA)	(20)	rat		997	Reagan & Becci (1985d)
ethyl chrysanthemate	-	rat		> 4640	Stauffer Chemical Co.(1984)

[a] Toxicity for male mice, 24 h after intraperitoneal injection or oral administration.
[b] Chemical identification numbers used in Table 1 and Fig. 2.

The same authors fed groups of 6 Long-Evans rats of each sex resmethrin in the diet at concentrations of 0, 61-90, 148-180, 297-386, 584-669, 1080-1375, or 1266-2532 mg/kg body weight per day for 14 days. Mortality was observed in the groups fed 1080 mg/kg or more. Tremor was observed at levels of 386 mg/kg or more (females only at 386 mg/kg). The terminal body weight and food utilization were significantly lower in the groups fed 1080 mg/kg or more compared with the controls. A significant increase in the hepatic organ-to-body weight ratios was noted at levels of 297 mg/kg or more. Compound-related histopathological changes were not observed in any of the tissues and organs examined. The maximum no-observed-adverse-effect dietary level was 148 mg/kg body weight per day for male and 180 mg/kg body weight per day for female rats (Swentzel et al., 1977).

In a third study by Swentzel et al. (1977), groups of 8-20 Long-Evans rats of each sex were fed resmethrin in the diet at concentrations equivalent to 0, 22, 66, 211, or 679 mg/kg body weight per day for males and of 0, 3, 7, 22, 67, 219, 724, or 2400 mg/kg body weight per day for females, for 90 days. All the females fed the highest level died. Tremor was observed at levels of 679 mg/kg or more. The mean terminal body weight was significantly lower in the group given 679-724 mg/kg than in the control group. A significant increase in the hepatic and renal organ-to-body weight ratios was noted in males fed 211 or 679 mg/kg; while, in females fed 219 or 724 mg/kg, only an increase in the hepatic ratio was observed. No significant differences were observed in clinical chemistry values (serum glutamic oxaloacetic transaminase (SGOT), serum glutamic pyruvic transaminase (SGPT), total lactate dehydrogenase (LDH), alkaline phosphatase (AP), gamma-glutamyl transpeptidase (GGTP), total bilirubin, total protein, blood-urea nitrogen (BUN)) between test and control animals. Compound-related histopathological changes were not observed in any of the tissues and organs examined. The maximum no-observed-adverse-effect dietary level was 67 mg/kg body weight per day for female and 66 mg/kg body weight per day for male rats.

Groups of rats (10 males/group) were administered bioresmethrin orally by gavage, daily, 6 days/week for 3 weeks at doses of 0, 1000, or 2000 mg/kg body weight. Body weights were slightly reduced at 2000 mg/kg. A slight reduction was noted in haemoglobin content and hematocrit value. Biochemical examination revealed an increase in albumin and blood-urea nitrogen concentrations and a decrease in serum-glutamic oxaloacetic transaminase (SGOT) activity. Increased liver size and reduced thymus weight were observed at 1000 mg/kg. Reduced prostate weight was noted only at the high dose. Histopathological examination revealed thymic involution (Glomot, unpublished report).[a]

Wallwork et al. (1971) reported a study in which groups of rats (18 males and 18 females/group) were fed bioresmethrin in the diet at concentrations of 0, 400, 1200, or 8000 mg/kg over 91 days. The group receiving the highest dose was fed 4000 mg/kg for 30 days and thereafter 8000 mg/kg. Body weights were reduced at the highest dose level and there were changes in blood chemistry parameters indicating liver dysfunction (an increase in serum-alkaline phosphatase (SAP), SGOT, and urinary nitrogen and a decrease in glucose content). The red blood cell count was depressed in the group receiving 1200 mg/kg. An increase in liver weight and a decrease in the weights of several other organs, such as the spleen and thymus, were observed at 4000 mg/kg. Fatty infiltration of the liver was noticed at 1200, 4000, and 8000 mg/kg. The no-observed-adverse-effect level in this study was 400 mg/kg, equivalent to an average daily intake of 32.8 and 36.1 mg/kg body weight for males and females, respectively.

Bioresmethrin was administered to groups of dogs (2 of each sex/group) by gavage, daily, at dose levels of 0 or 500 mg/kg for 7 days followed by an increased dose of 1000 mg/kg for a further 14 days. No effects were noted on mortality, behaviour, body weight, haematology, blood chemistry, urinalysis, or electrocardiograms (Malone & Chesher, 1970).

Groups of dogs (3 males and 3 females/group) were administered bioresmethrin in gelatin capsule by gavage, daily for 90 days, at dosage levels of 0, 25, 80, or 250 mg/kg body weight (the highest dose was increased to 500 mg/kg body weight in week 7). There were no effects on mortality, body weight, food consumption, ophthalmology, or urinalysis. Red blood cell count, haemoglobin content, and packed cell volume values were reduced at the highest dose level. Blood-urea nitrogen was slightly increased at the highest dose after 12 weeks. No adverse effects were observed on gross or histopathological examination. The no-observed-adverse-effect level was 80 mg/kg body weight, equivalent to an average of 1600 mg/kg diet (Noel et al., 1971).

In summary, the no-observed-adverse-effect level for resmethrin as determined in the 90-day study on rats was 66 mg/kg body weight per day, whereas that for bioresmethrin was 33 mg/kg body weight per day in the 91-day study on rats and 80 mg/kg body weight per day in the 90-day study on dogs.

---

[a] GLOMOT, R. (undated) Etude de la toxicité chronique de 3 semaines chez le rat du RU11484 (NRDC 107) (Unpublished report of Roussel Uclaf submitted to WHO by Wellcome Foundation Ltd).

7.2.2 Inhalation

Short-term inhalation studies were performed using three resmethrin formulations and one blank formulation. Aerosol spray formulations (frequency median diameter of the particles: 1.5-2.0 µm, volume median diameter 10-18.5 µm) were introduced into the top of a pyramid-shaped sealed chamber and dispersed for 30-second intervals every 30 min. Groups of 25 male rats, 10 female rats, and 4 male rabbits were exposed to the inhalations 10 times a day, over a period of 5 h, for 5 consecutive days. Daily active ingredient concentrations of each formulation in the chamber were 2.9-3.2 mg/litre, based on the weight loss from each spray can. The clinical signs included increased preening, ruffled pelt, rapid breathing, and slight nasal discharge. All signs disappeared overnight, but recurred after each daily exposure. In rats, there were no effects on body weight. No gross or histopathological lesions related to exposure to the formulations were observed in rats necropsied immediately after the last 5-h exposure and 7 and 14 days after exposure. No indication of toxic effects, other than irritation, was observed in any test (Macko et al., 1979).

When ICR mice and Sprague-Dawley rats were exposed to [1R, trans, cis]-resmethrin (at concentrations of 0, 23, 47, or 210 mg/m^3) for 4 h/day, 5 days/week over 4 weeks, no toxic effects were observed on behaviour, food intake, haematology, clinical biochemistry, mortality, or histopathology (Miyamoto, 1976).

When groups of 16 male and 16 female Wistar rats were exposed through inhalation for 6 h/day on 5 days of each week, over a period of 90 days, to technical resmethrin at target exposure levels of 0.1, 0.3, or 1.0 g/m^3, the no-observed-adverse-effect level was established at 0.1 g/m^3. At 0.3 g/m^3, there were minor effects on some clinical pathology parameters and also signs of irritation. However, microscopic pathological examination did not reveal any treatment-related changes in the lungs or other organs of rats exposed at this level. At 1 g/m^3, there were clinical signs indicative of irritation, minor neurobehavioural changes, a reduced rate of weight gain, and some changes in clinical pathology parameters. Microscopic examination at this level showed minimal changes in the larynx, liver, and thyroid, but these were reversible during the recovery period. There were no treatment-related lung changes (Coombs et al., 1985).

7.2.3 Dermal application

Resmethrin was applied twice a week for 3 weeks to the shaved skin of 4 groups of 10 male New Zealand White rabbits.

Cotton cloth treated with resmethrin at 0.247 mg/cm³ was applied over 1 ml of liquid (imitating sweat) to rabbits in the first group. In the second group, cotton cloth treated with resmethrin was applied without the sweat, and in the third group, the cotton cloth was fixed to skin that had been pretreated with 10 g of technical grade resmethrin. In the fourth group, untreated cotton cloth was fixed over skin pretreated with pyrax powder containing 1% resmethrin at the rate of 1 g/kg of body weight. The 3 control groups received cotton cloth treated with acetone, cotton cloth treated with acetone over 1 ml of the sweat, and untreated cotton cloth over 1 g pyrax powder/kg, respectively. No significant changes were noted, on day 24 of the test, in rabbit body weights and organ-to-body weight ratios of liver, lung, kidney, testis, and spleen. Average dermal irritation scores for resmethrin-treated rabbits were not significantly higher than those for the control groups and did not increase during the test. No significant trends compared with the controls were seen in clinical chemistry values (serum-glutamic oxaloacetic transaminase, serum-glutamic pyruvic transaminase, lactic dehydrogenase, alkaline phosphatase, blood-urea nitrogen) on days 5, 12, 19, and 24 of the test. There were no compound-related lesions of the skin or of any of the other tissues and organs examined at the termination of the study (Swentzel et al., 1977).

7.3 Primary Irritation and Sensitization

Technical grade resmethrin was found to be a slight irritant in rabbits in a 24 day dorsal/ventral rabbit ear test. Dermal irritation was evident on both intact and abraded skin at 72 h and up to 7 days. Resmethrin did not cause sensitization reactions in guinea-pigs, or photochemical irritation in New Zealand White rabbits. Repeated daily applications of 0.1 g of the technical grade compound to one ear of each of 5 New Zealand White rabbits were carried out for 30 consecutive days as well as applications of compound-impregnated cotton sateen cloth (0.247 mg/cm²) with artificial sweat for 24 days. In this study, resmethrin did not produce acne-form dermatitis (Swentzel et al., 1977).

Groups of adult guinea-pigs (6 males/group) were treated with bioresmethrin (0.1 ml of a 5% (w/v) formulation) or 2,4-dinitrochloro benzene (DNCB) (0.1 ml of a 1% (w/v) formulation in mineral oil) to assess the sensitization properties. The test substance was applied to the ears for 4 days. On day 7, 0.2 ml was applied dermally and the degree of irritation recorded. As expected, the DNCB was an irritant while bioresmethrin showed only traces of erythema suggesting a low potential for sensitization and irritation (Chesher & Malone, 1970b).

Instillation of technical bioresmethrin into the eye of 6 rabbits (0.1 ml) did not produce any irritation or corneal damage, or any indication of ocular hazard (Chesher & Malone, 1970c).

7.4 Long-term Exposure and Carcinogenicity

When [1R, trans, cis]-resmethrin was fed to Sprague-Dawley rats (male and female) at dietary levels of 500, 1500, or 5000 mg/kg for 24 weeks, toxic symptoms, such as tremors and decreased body weight, increased liver and kidney weights and an increase in alkaline phosphatase activity were observed at 5000 mg/kg. The no-observed-adverse-effect level was 1500 mg/kg (77.7 mg/kg per day for males and 86.6 mg/kg per day for females) (Miyamoto, 1976).

Resmethrin fed to Wistar rats at dosage levels of 0, 500, 2500, or 5000 mg/kg in the basal diet over a 112-week period, was determined not to be oncogenic up to, and including, 5000 mg/kg, which was the highest dose tested. The no-observed-adverse-effect level of 500 mg/kg for toxic effects, was the lowest effect level for hypertrophy of hepatocytes, which was not considered a definite toxic response (Knickerbocker et al., 1980; Hess et al., 1982).

Cox et al. (1979a) fed CD-1 outbred albino mice with 0, 250, 500, or 1000 mg resmethrin/kg basal diet for an 85-week period. No oncogenicity was observed at any doses up to and including 1000 mg/kg.

When Beagle dogs were administered 0, 10, 30, or 300 mg resmethrin/kg body weight for 6 months, the no-observed-adverse-effect level was 10 mg/kg per day. On day 57 of the study, the highest dose level was increased from 100 mg/kg per day to 300 mg/kg per day. Increased liver weights were noted at 30 mg/kg body weight per day (Gephart et al., 1980).

An acceptable daily intake (ADI) was established by the USA EPA at 0.125 mg/kg body weight per day based on no-observed-adverse-effect levels in long-term toxicity studies. A food additive tolerance has been established by the US EPA, permitting resmethrin residues of up to 3 ppm, in or on food commodities, resulting from use in food handling areas (US Environmental Protection Agency, 1983).

7.5 Mutagenicity

Saccharomyces cerevisiae D4 and five strains of *Salmonella typhimurium* (TA1535, TA1537, TA1538, TA98, and TA100) were used to evaluate the mutagenic potential of resmethrin. The compound was tested in the absence or presence of liver microsomal enzyme preparations from rats pre-treated with Aroclor 1254. Resmethrin was not mutagenic to any of the indicator organisms under both conditions (Swentzel et al., 1977).

Resmethrin, bioresmethrin, and cismethrin were tested for mutagenicity in several test systems. Miyamoto (1976) and Suzuki (1975) used the *Escherichia coli* and *S.typhimurium* reverse mutation tests. Garret et al. (1986) summarized results of point/gene mutations in prokaryotes or eukaryotes, primary DNA damage in prokaryotes or eukaryotes, chromosomal effects in Chinese hamster ovary cells, mouse bone marrow, and cardiac blood cells of the mouse. Pluijmen et al. (1984) used reverse mutation tests in *S.typhimurium* TA98 or TA100, or mutagenicity tests with V79 Chinese hamster cells to test seven synthetic pyrethroids including resmethrin, bioresmethrin, and cismethrin. They all gave negative results.

Bioresmethrin was also tested in a metaphase chromosome analysis of cultured human lymphocytes, an autoradiographic assessment of unscheduled DNA synthesis in mammalian cells, and a mouse micronucleus test. They also gave negative results (Allen et al., 1986; Allen & Proudlock, 1986; Vannier & Fournex, 1986).

7.6 Reproductive effects, Embryotoxicity, and Teratogenicity

Three groups of 30 pregnant Long-Evans rats were administered resmethrin in the diet at concentrations of 0, 188, or 1500 mg/kg from day 6 to day 16 of gestation. The dams showed tremors and decreased food and water consumption at 1500 mg/kg and 2 dams died; the lower fetal weight seen at this dose and the resorption of embryos and fetuses in 15 out of 30 dams were probably due to maternal toxicity. No gross abnormalities of fetal skeletons and soft tissues were observed in the treated groups. Thus, the consumption of resmethrin in ground feed was not teratogenic at 188 and 1500 mg/kg (Swentzel et al., 1977).

In a 3-generation study, Sprague-Dawley rats were fed resmethrin in the diet at 0, 500, 800, or 1250 mg/kg (Schwartz et al., 1979c). A slight increase in the number of pups cast dead and a decrease in pup weights were noted at the 500 mg/kg level. A no-observed-adverse-effect level of < 500 mg/kg was established for pups cast dead and reduced pup weights at 21 days.

Sprague-Dawley female albino rats were given resmethrin in corn oil, by gavage, at dose levels of 0, 20, 40, or 80 mg/kg during the period of major organogenesis (days 6-15 of gestation). Resmethrin was not teratogenic in rats at levels up to, and including, 80 mg/kg. The no-observed-adverse-effect level for fetotoxicity was 40 mg/kg (Machi et al., 1979).

Pregnant New Zealand White Minnikin rabbits were given resmethrin by oral intubation at 0, 10, 30, or 100 mg/kg body weight per day on days 6-18 of gestation (Becci et al., 1979). On day 29 of gestation, all animals were killed for examination. No teratogenic effects were seen at dose levels up to and including 100 mg/kg.

When [1R, trans, cis]-resmethrin was administered orally to female ICR mice (10, 30, or 100 mg/kg, daily) and Sprague-Dawley rats (10, 20, or 50 mg/kg daily) during the period of gestation, to examine maternal and embryotoxic effects, no significant adverse effects, such as abortion, resorption of fetuses or embryos, external or skeletal abnormalities of pups, and abnormalities in growth or organ differentiation, were observed at any doses (Miyamoto, 1976).

Groups of pregnant rabbits (4-6 rabbits/group) were administered bioresmethrin at doses of 0, 10, 20, 40, or 80 mg/kg, by gavage, daily, from day 8 to day 16 of gestion. The does were sacrificed on day 28 and examined for implantation, live and dead fetuses, resorption sites, and abnormalities. There was no apparent effect on parents in the study as growth and gestation were unaffected. There was an increase in the numbers of dead fetuses at the highest dose and a large number of resorption sites were noted at all treatment levels. A number of deformed fetuses were observed, but the total numbers were not sufficient for an adequate statistical evaluation. The deformities included straight tail, crossed hind limbs, and unilateral union of 6th and 7th ribs at the sternal end. An overall fetal loss was observed at all dose levels (primarily because of the large number of resorption sites recorded) (Waldron, 1969).

7.7 Immunotoxicity

The influence of various pesticides on the humoral and cellular immune response to fluorescein-labelled ovalbumin has been analysed. Resmethrin was administered intragastrically in corn oil as a single dose (one half of LD_{50}) before primary immunization. Control groups included animals treated with corn oil alone, or immunosuppressed with methotrexate. Booster immunizations and test bleedings were scheduled to follow at weekly intervals. The cellular immune response was quantified by redness and swelling, histological examination, and by differential temperature measurements of the foot pads after antigen challenge. The concentration, binding affinity, and heterogeneity of the serum antibody were determined by fluorescence polarization measurements. Resmethrin gave an early, sometimes very marked, stimulation of the cellular immune response (Danliker et al., 1979).

7.8 Neurotoxicity

The neurotoxicity of resmethrin was evaluated in three short-term dietary studies on Sprague-Dawley rats designed to examine the gross and histopathological changes to the central and peripheral nervous system. Resmethrin was not neurotoxic when administered at 1250 mg/kg for 32 weeks, 5000 mg/kg for 30 days, or 12 640 mg/kg for 7 days (Cox et al., 1979b; Schwartz et al., 1979a,b).

In order to better characterize the behavioural effects of pyrethroid insecticides, comparisons were made of the effects of cismethrin and deltamethrin exposure on motor activity and the acoustic startle response in male Long-Evans rats (Crofton & Reiter, 1984). Acute dose effect, acute time course, and 30-day repeated-exposure determinations of 1 h motor activity were made using figure-eight mazes. The acoustic startle response to a 13-kHz, 120-dB, 40-msecond tone was measured at each of three background white noise levels (50, 65, and 80 dB). Deltamethrin (0, 2, 4, 6, or 8 mg/kg) or cismethrin (0, 6, 12, 18, or 24 mg/kg) was administered orally in 0.2 ml corn oil/kg. Both compounds produced similar dose-dependent decreases in motor activity. The time course of onset and recovery for this decreased activity was rapid (1-4 h). No cumulative effects on motor activity were found of a 30-day exposure to 2 mg deltamethrin/kg per day or 6 mg cismethrin/kg per day. The effects of cismethrin and deltamethrin on the acoustic startle response differed. Deltamethrin produced a dose-dependent decrease in amplitude and an increase in latency, and cismethrin produced an increase in amplitude and no change in latency. The differential effects of cismethrin (Type I pyrethroids) and deltamethrin (Type II pyrethroids) on the acoustic startle response may be related to the contrasting effects previously shown with neurophysiological and/or neurochemical techniques (see Annex).

The isolated rat neurohypophysis, which shows a calcium-dependent hormone release when depolarized in vitro, was used as a model system to investigate the effects of the pyrethroids deltamethrin and resmethrin on mammalian nervous tissue (Dyball, 1982). Both compounds inhibited neurohypophysial hormone release in response to electrical stimulation, deltamethrin being more potent than resmethrin. Deltamethrin reduced the hormone content of the neurohypophysis. Resmethrin did not reduce stored hormone significantly and its effects on release were dose dependent. They could be mimicked by raising the Na^+ of the medium, but not by lowering the Ca^{2+}. Resmethrin did not have any effects on the release of hormone following depolarization of the tissue with a raised K^+. The results are consistent with the suggestion that the compounds do not act on the potential-dependent secretion process but rather on the mechanism linking depolarization of the secretory terminals with the arrival of action potentials, possibly by interfering with sodium-channel activation and inactivation.

The neurological effects of four synthetic pyrethroids resmethrin, permethrin, cypermethrin, and deltamethrin were investigated in the rat to establish whether there is a correlation between the clinical-functional status of the animal and peripheral nerve damage, as measured biochemically (Rose & Dewar, 1983). Neuromuscular dysfunction was assessed by means of the inclined plane test and peripheral nerve damage by reference to β-glucuronidase and β-galactosidase activity increases in nerve tissue homogenates from treated and control animals. A transient functional impairment was found in animals treated with any one of the four pyrethroids tested and, in all cases, this was maximal at the end of the 7-day dosing regimen (resmethrin doses of 500-2000 mg/kg per day). Significant increases in β-glucuronidase and β-galactosidase were found, 3-4 weeks after the start of dosing in the distal portion of the sciatic/posterior tibial nerves of animals treated with permethrin, cypermethrin, or deltamethrin; however, no changes were found in resmethrin-treated animals. Thus, it is concluded that there is no direct correlation between the time-course of the neuromuscular dysfunction and the neurobiochemical changes. This suggests that these pyrethroids have at least two distinct actions, a short-term pharmacological effect and, at near-lethal dose levels, a more chronic neurotoxic effect that results in sparse axonal nerve damage.

Resmethrin (30 µmol/litre)-induced release of transmitters was not affected by manipulation of the Na^+ current with either choline or tetrodotoxin agents, which readily reversed the effects of veratridine, deltamethrin, and cypermethrin (Doherty et al., 1986). Resmethrin (I_{50}: 2.2 µmol/litre) inhibited the ATP-dependent uptake of Ca^{2+} but deltamethrin and cypermethrin were much less effective. Resmethrin also displaced Ca^{2+} from crude synaptosomal membranes. The release-promoting effects of resmethrin in rat brain *in vitro* are better explained by its effects on Ca^{2+} rather than by a specific effect on the Na^+ channel. In contrast, deltamethrin and cypermethrin promote transmitter release by a Na^+ dependent process.

Glickman & Casida (1982) discussed species and structural variations affecting pyrethroid neurotoxicity. They concluded that the mammalian nervous system, or at least the brain, appears to lack sites sensitive to bioresmethrin and to a lesser extent to [1R, trans]-permethrin, yet small structural changes restore the toxicity (e.g., [1R,trans]-ethano-resmethrin and [1R, cis]-resmethrin. The authors reported that birds and mammals in general respond to *cis*- but not to *trans*-resmethrin in contrast to insects, crustaceans, and fish, which are highly sensitive to both isomers. Furthermore, common green lacewing larvae are very tolerant to pyrethroids, suggesting possible involvement of nerve insensitivity in addition to detoxification in this species. These examples of insensitivity may be associated with modified sites of action or perhaps an increased stabilization of nerve membranes making them more resistant to pyrethroid-induced excitation.

7.9 Mechanism of Toxicity (Mode of Action)

Cismethrin is toxic for both insects and mammals. Bioresmethrin is about 50 times less toxic than cismethrin and produces few symptoms in mice and rats, even at extremely high doses. The poisoning syndrome of cismethrin and bioresmethrin was characterized by whole body tremors (T-syndrome) and both compounds were therefore classified as Type I pyrethroids (Verschoyle & Aldridge, 1980; Lawrence & Casida, 1982, Annex).

Tremors started when the concentrations of cismethrin and bioresmethrin in the brain were 0.5-1 mg/kg and 4-5 mg/kg, respectively. At death, brain levels of cismethrin were 3.9-5.1 mg/kg, and those of bioresmethrin were 23-35 mg/kg. As liver microsomal esterases hydrolysed bioresmethrin 10 times more rapidly than cismethrin, the lower toxicity of bioresmethrin was partly attributed to its faster metabolism and intrinsically lower toxicity at the critical site of action in the nervous system (White et al., 1976).

Cismethrin given intravenously produced repetitive activity, after external stimulation, in the spinal cord of rabbit (Carlton, 1977). As γ-aminobutyric acid (GABA) blockers, such as bicuculline and picrotoxin, produced convulsions similar to those of cismethrin, the effects of the compounds on dorsal root potentials were examined in the rat. Bicuculline reduced the amplitude of the potential to 67% of the control values, but cismethrin enhanced the potential to 142% of the control values. The convulsions associated with cismethrin poisoning, therefore, are not produced by an antagonism of GABA-mediated inhibitory transmission (Smith, 1980).

Administration of cismethrin into the lateral ventricle of the brain or into the spinal cord causes signs similar to those observed after intravenous administration. The onset of tremors after intraventricular administration of cismethrin was delayed for about 15 min while, after intraspinal injection, the symptoms occurred within 2-5 min, indicating that cismethrin may act directly on the spinal cord rather than in the brain (Gray et al., 1980b).

After intravenous administration of [^{14}C]-alcohol-labelled cismethrin or bioresmethrin to rats, the parent pyrethroid was rapidly cleared from the blood and liver, and both isomers rapidly entered the central nervous system (CNS) reaching peak concentrations within 2-5 min. Cismethrin concentrations in the brain exceeding 3.5 nmol/g were associated only with animals showing tremors. These levels of cismethrin were maintained for up to 30 min, but bioresmethrin was depleted more rapidly, possibly due to brain metabolism. It is concluded that the low toxicity of bioresmethrin is possibly because of its inability to interact with the site of action in the CNS and to its rapid metabolism in the liver (Gray et al., 1980a).

Cismethrin produced repetitive firing in the flight muscles and uncoupling of motor unit activity in the housefly (Miller & Adams, 1977), and repetitive firing in a cercal sensory nerve of the cockroach (Gammon et al., 1981). On the basis of the electrophysiological effects and symptomatology in insects as well as in mammals, cismethrin is classified as a Type I pyrethroid, characterized by a mainly peripheral nervous system action (Gammon et al., 1981).

7.10 Potentiation

Groups of rats (6 female rats/group) were administered bioresmethrin, bioallethrin, and/or piperonyl butoxide, alone or in combinations, at doses approximating the acute intraperitoneal LD_{50} value. No potentiation of the acute toxicity was observed in this study. In all cases with bioresmethrin combinations, the observed LD_{50} values were equal to, or exceeded, the expected value (Wallwork & Malone, 1971).

8. EFFECTS ON MAN

Although the resmethrins have been used for many years, no data have been reported on their toxicity for human beings.

9. EVALUATION OF HUMAN HEALTH RISKS AND EFFECTS ON THE ENVIRONMENT

9.1 Human Health Risks

Resmethrin, consisting of four stereo-isomers, is an effective insecticide mainly used to control household insects and other public health insects, with applications in the food handling and storage areas.

Bioresmethrin and cismethrin are composed of a selected isomer(s). As with resmethrin, bioresmethrin is used to control household insects and other public health insects. In addition, bioresmethrin is used as a post-harvest insecticide to control stored grain pest. Human exposure to the resmethrins will be mainly via inhalation, when the formulations are sprayed in the form of a mist, though the use in food handling and storage areas as well as post-harvest treatment may result in dietary residues. Air levels following conventional household aerosol spraying with the resmethrins are not expected to exceed 0.5 mg/m^3.

The only significant potential dietary exposure will result from the use of resmethrin on stored grain. Residues of up to 4 mg/kg might be present in grain, but this would be reduced to zero in white bread. However, reduced residues may be present in wholemeal bread. A food additive tolerance has been established by the US Environmental Protection Agency (US EPA) permitting resmethrin residues of up to 3 mg/kg (3 ppm), in or on food commodities, resulting from use in food handling areas. An ADI was established by the US EPA at 0.1250 mg/kg body weight per day, based on no-observed-adverse-effect levels in long-term toxicity studies. No data are available on occupational exposure to the resmethrins. Although the resmethrins have been used for many years, no data have been reported concerning their toxicity for human beings. Thus, to determine the potential toxicity for human beings, extrapolation from animal data and in vitro studies has been used.

The result of short-term studies on experimental animals suggest that resmethrins are weakly toxic when administered by various routes of exposure (oral LD_{50} of resmethrin: 690 mg/kg (mouse) - > 5000 mg/kg (rat); those of bioresmethrin: 225 mg/kg (rabbit), 480-10 000 mg/kg (mouse), 8800 mg/kg (rats)). Cismethrin showed moderate toxicity for the mouse (oral LD_{50} 152-160 mg/kg). The acute toxicity of resmethrin metabolites were in the same range in the rat, but somewhat more toxic in the mouse.

While technical grade resmethrin is a slight skin irritant, it is not a sensitizer.

Resmethrins are not mutagenic in a variety of test systems, including gene mutations, DNA damage and DNA repair, and chromosomal effects.

Resmethrin was not carcinogenic for mice or rats, when fed at dietary levels of up to 1000 mg/kg for 85 weeks and 5000 mg/kg for 112 weeks, respectively.

Resmethrin was not teratogenic in the rat, mouse, or rabbit, up to dose levels of 100 mg/kg body weight. A level of 40 mg/kg body weight appeared to be the no-observed-adverse-effect level for fetotoxicity in the rat.

Resmethrins at near lethal doses are likely to cause hyperactivity, tremors, and convulsions and have been classified as Type I pyrethroids.

For resmethrin, a no-observed-adverse-effect level was established in a 90-day rat study to be 66-67 mg/kg body weight per day, whereas, in another 2-year rat study, the lowest effect level appeared to be 500 mg/kg diet, corresponding to 25 mg/kg body weight per day. In a 6-month feeding study on dogs, the no-observed-adverse-effect level was 10 mg/kg body weight per day.

In a 90-day inhalation study on rats, a no-observed-adverse-effect level was established of 0.1 g/m^3.

The no-observed-adverse-effect level for bioresmethrin in a 9-day feeding study on the rat was 33-36 mg/kg body weight per day; and in a 90-day study on dogs, it was 80 mg/kg body weight per day.

In a 24-week feeding study on rats, the no-observed-adverse-effect level for [1R, trans, cis]-resmethrin was 1500 mg/kg diet corresponding to 75 mg/kg body weight.

9.2 Effects on the Environment

Resmethrins are used mainly indoors for the control of household insects and also for stored grain protection. They are also used in greenhouses and can be used outdoors for mosquito control. However, under outdoor conditions, rapid photodegradation and microbial degradation in the soil ensure that residues will not persist to any extent in the environment.

In laboratory studies, resmethrins have been shown to be very toxic for fish (96-h LC_{50} values: 0.3-5.5 µg/litre) but less toxic for *Daphnia* and aquatic insect larvae. However, under field conditions the low water solubility of the resmethrins and their ready degradation greatly alleviate the effects that might be predicted from the laboratory studies. The toxicity of resmethrins for birds is low (LD_{50} > 5000 mg/kg) and they do not produce any effects on avian reproduction.

10. CONCLUSIONS

General population: Under recommended conditions of household and other public health use, the exposure of the general population to resmethrins is negligible and is unlikely to present a hazard. Under recommended conditions of use in food handling and storage areas as well as in post-harvest treatment, the exposure of the general population to resmethrins in the diet is unlikely to exceed the ADI established by the US EPA.

Occupational exposure: With reasonable work practices, hygienic measures, and safety precautions, the use of resmethrins is unlikely to present a hazard to those occupationally exposed to it.

Environment: With recommended application rates, it is unlikely that resmethrins or their degradation products will attain levels of environmental significance. In spite of the fact that resmethrins are highly toxic for fish, this is only likely to cause a problem in the case of spillage or over-spraying.

11. RECOMMENDATIONS

- In order to fully assess the potential dietary exposure from current uses of resmethrins, it is suggested that the degradation pathway on stored grain be studied, and the terminal residues on grain and bread be defined.

- It is considered that resmethrin, despite its high octanol-water partition coefficient, is very unlikely to bioaccumulate in non-target species, because of its ready degradation. However, experimental confirmation of this in fish might be useful.

- A further multigeneration reproduction study to define a no-observed-adverse-effect level should be considered.

- Over many years of use, no adverse effects have been reported as a result of human exposure to resmethrins, but it is still necessary to maintain observations on human exposure.

- The labelling of resmethrins for household use should include adequate instructions for use and storage and, where appropriate, a warning of flammability.

- Efforts should be made to obtain a more precise estimate of the total global usage of resmethrins.

12. PREVIOUS EVALUATION BY INTERNATIONAL BODIES

The Joint FAO/WHO Expert Committee on Pesticide Residues (JMPR) discussed and evaluated bioresmethrin at its meetings in 1975 and 1976 (FAO/WHO, 1976, 1977). An acceptable daily intake (ADI) has not been established.

The Pesticide Development and Safe Use Unit, Division of Vector Biology and Control, WHO, has classified bioresmethrin as a technical product unlikely to present an acute hazard in normal use, and resmethrin and cismethrin as slightly hazardous (WHO, 1986). A Data Sheet on bioresmethrin (No. 34) has been issued (WHO/FAO, 1978).

REFERENCES

ABBOTT, D.D. (1971) Total degradation products of SBP-1382. Acute oral LD50/mice, 6 pp (Unpublished proprietary data supplied by Roussel Uclaf).

ABE, Y., TSUDA, K., & FUJITA, Y. (1972) Studies on pyrethroidal compounds. Part III. Photostability of pyrethroidal compounds. Botyu-Kagaku, 37: 102-110.

ALLEN, J.A. & PROUDLOCK, R.J. (1986) Autoradiographic assessment of unscheduled DNA repair synthesis in mammalian cells after exposure to bioresmethrin, Huntington, United Kingdom, Huntingdon Research Centre, 18 pp (Report No. RSL-BRM-698/851420/A) (Unpublished proprietary data supplied by Roussel Uclaf).

ALLEN, J.A., BROOKER, P.C., & HOWELL, A. (1986) Bioresmethrin metaphase chromosome analysis of human lymphocytes cultures in vitro, Huntingdon, United Kingdom, Huntingdon Research Centre, 15 pp (Report No. RSL-BRM-697/851370/A) (Unpublished proprietary data supplied by Roussel Uclaf).

ARDLEY J.H. (1975) Report of milling and baking trials with bioresmethrin treated wheat (Unpublished report of Wellcome Australia Ltd).

BAKER, P.G. & BOTTOMLEY, P. (1982) Determination of residues of synthetic pyrethroids in fruit and vegetables by gas-liquid and high-performance liquid chromatography. Analyst, 107: 206-212.

BATTELLE (1982) Pesticide programme of research and market planning. Part I: Insecticides, Geneva, Battelle Institute.

BECCI, P.J., KNICKERBOCKER, M., & PARENT, R.A. (1979) Teratological evaluation of SBP-1382 in albino rabbits, Waverly, New York, Food and Drug Research Laboratories, 17 pp (Report No. 6288) (Unpublished proprietary data supplied by Roussel Uclaf).

BENGSTON, M., COOPER, L.M., & GRANT-TAYLOR, F.J. (1975) A comparison of bioresmethrin, chlorpyrifos-methyl and pirimiphos-methyl as grain protectants against malathion-resistant insects in wheat. Queensland J. Agric. anim. Sci., 32: 51-78.

BUICK, A.R. & FLANAGAN, P. (1973) The fate of NRDC 107 (bioresmethrin) on tomatoes (Report No. HEGH 73/1) (Unpublished data of Wellcome Foundation Ltd).

BURT, M.E. (1983a) Resmethrin residues in tomato and cucumber, New Brunswick, Rutgers State University of New Jersey, Agricultural Experiment Station, 18 pp (Unpublished proprietary data supplied by Roussel Uclaf).

BURT, M.E. (1983b) Resmethrin residues in lettuce (greenhouse), New Brunswick, Rutgers State University of New Jersey, Agricultural Experiment Station, 18 pp (Unpublished proprietary data supplied by Roussel Uclaf).

CARLTON, M. (1977) Some effects of cismethrin on the rabbit nervous system. Pestic. Sci., 8: 700-712.

CAVE, S.L. (1981) Simultaneous estimation of bioresmethrin and piperonylbutoxide by gas-liquid chromatography with chemical-ionization mass spectrometry. Pestic. Sci., 12: 156-160.

CHAPMAN, R.A. & HARRIS, C.R. (1978) Extraction and liquid-solid chromatography cleanup procedures for the direct analysis of four pyrethroid insecticides in crops by gas-liquid chromatography. J. Chromatogr., 166: 513-518.

CHESHER, B.C. & MALONE, J.C. (1970a) Acute toxicity tests with NRDC 107 in hens (Report No. B 236-70) (Unpublished data of Wellcome Foundation Ltd).

CHESHER, B.C. & MALONE, J.C. (1970b) Sensitisation study with NRDC 107 on guinea pigs (Report B 198-70) (Unpublished data of Wellcome Foundation Ltd).

CHESHER, B.C. & MALONE, J.C. (1970c) Ocular irritancy of NRDC 107 in rabbits (Report No. B 217-70) (Unpublished data of Wellcome Foundation Ltd).

CHESHER, B.C. & MALONE, J.C. (1971a) Toxicity to dogs of NRDC 107 (continuation) (Report No. B 27-71) (Unpublished data of Wellcome Foundation Ltd).

CHESHER B.C. & MALONE J.C. (1971b) Acute toxicity of NRDC 107 by the intravenous route. (Report No. B 329-71) (Unpublished data of Wellcome Foundation Ltd).

CHRISTOPHER, R.J., MUNGER, C.E., & WAYNE IRVIE, G. (1985) Distribution and depletion of [^{14}C]-resmethrin isomers administered orally to laying hens. Pestic. Sci., 16: 378-382.

COOMBS, D.W., HARDY, C.J., CLARK, G.C., STREET, A.E., GOPINATH, C., LEWIS, D.J., & RAO, R.S. (1985) Resmethrin 90-day inhalation toxicity study in the rat, Huntingdon, United Kingdom, Huntingdon Research Centre, 80 pp (Report No. SBP 6/84997) (Unpublished proprietary data supplied by Roussel Uclaf).

COX, G.E., KNICKERBOCKER, M., & PARENT, R.A. (1979a) Evaluation of dietary administration of SBP-1382 in CD-1 outbred albino mice over an 85-week period, Waverly, New York, Food and Drug Research Laboratories, 52 pp (Report No. 5270) (Unpublished proprietary data supplied by Roussel Uclaf).

COX, G.E., BECCI, P.J., & PARENT, R.A. (1979b) Supplementary report for evaluation of the neurotoxic effects of SBP-1382 in albino rats - phase I, Waverly, New York, Food and Drug Research Laboratories, 7 pp (Report No. 6362) (Unpublished proprietary data supplied by Roussel Uclaf).

CROFTON, K.M. & REITER, L.W. (1984) Effects of two pyrethroid insecticides on motor activity and the acoustic startle response in the rat. Toxicol. appl. Pharmacol., 75: 318-328.

DANLIKER, W.B., HICKS, A.N., LEVISON, S.A., STEWART, K., & BROWN, R.J. (1979) Effects of pesticides on immume response, Washington, DC, US Environmental Protection Agency (EPA-600/1-79-039-PB 80-1308 34).

DESMARCHELIER, J.M. (1980) Comparative study of analytical methods for bioresmethrin, phenothrin, d-phenothrin, pyrethrum I, carbaryl, fenitrothion, methacrifos, pirimifos-methyl and dichlorfos on various grains. J. Pestic. Sci., 5: 521-532.

DEVAUX, Ph. & BOLLA, P. (1986) Bioresmethrin n-octanol/water partition coefficient and water solubility, Romainville, France, Roussel Uclaf, 4 pp (Report No. RU-BRM-142.06.86. STE/A) (Unpublished proprietary data).

DEVAUX, Ph. & TILLIER, C. (1986) Vapor pressure of bio-allethrin and bioresmethrin, Romainville, France, Roussel Uclaf, 8 pp (Report No. RU-BRM/BA-150.06.86.STE/A) (Unpublished proprietary data).

DOHERTY, J.D., LAUTER, C.J., & SALEM, N., Jr (1986) Synaptic effects on the synthetic pyrethroid resmethrin in rat brain in vitro. Comp. Biochem. Physiol., C84: 373-379.

DYBALL, R.E.J. (1982) Inhibition by decamethrin and resmethrin of hormone release from the isolated rat neurohypophysis: A model mammalian neurosecretory system. Pestic. Biochem. Physiol., 17: 42-47.

ELLIOT, M. (1976) Properties and applications of pyrethroids. Environ. Health Perspect., 14: 3-13.

ELLIOTT, M. (1977) Synthetic pyrethroids, Washington, DC, American Chemical Society, p. 229 (ACS Symposium Series, No. 42).

ELLIOTT, M., FARNMAN, A.W., JONES, N.F., NEEDHAM, P.H., & PEARSON, B.C. (1967) 5-Benzyl-3-furylmethyl chrysanthemate: a new potent insecticide. Nature (Lond.), 213: 493-494.

EVANS, M.H. (1976) End-plate potentials in frog muscle exposed to a synthetic pyrethroid. Pestic. Biochem. Physiol., 6: 547-550.

FAO (1982) Second Government Consultation on International Harmonization of Pesticide Registration Requirements, Rome, 11-15 October, 1982, Rome, Food and Agriculture Organization of the United Nations.

FAO/WHO (1976) Bioresmethrin. In: 1975 Evaluation of some pesticide residues in food, Geneva, World Health Organization, pp. 17-40 (WHO Pesticide Residues Series, No. 5).

FAO/WHO (1977) Bioresmethrin. In: 1976 Evaluation of some pesticide residues in food, Rome, Food and Agriculture Organization of the United Nations, pp. 55-78 (AGP: 1976/M/14).

FLANNIGAN, S.A. & TUCKER, S.B. (1985) Variation in cutaneous sensation between synthetic pyrethroid insecticides. Contact Dermatitis, 13: 140-147.

GAINES, T.B. & LINDER, R.E. (1986) Acute toxicity of pesticides in adult and weanling rats. Fundam. appl. Toxicol., 7: 299-308.

GAMMON, D.W. & CASIDA, J.E. (1983) Pyrethroids of the most potent class antagonize GABA action at the crayfish neuromuscular junction. Neurosci. Lett., 40: 163-168.

GAMMON, D.W., BROWN, M.A., & CASIDA, J.E. (1981) Two classes of pyrethroid action in the cockroach. Pestic. Biochem. Physiol., 15: 181-191.

GAMMON, D.W., LAWRENCE, L.J., & CASIDA, J.E. (1982) Pyrethroid toxicology: Protective effects of Diazepam and phenobarbital in the mouse and the cockroach. Toxicol. appl. Pharmacol., 66: 290-296.

GARRET, N.E., FRANK STACK, H., & WATERS, D. (1986) Evaluation of the genetic activity profiles of 65 pesticides. Mutat. Res., 168: 301-325.

GEPHART, L.A., JOHNSON, W.D., BECCI, P.J., & PARENT, R.A. (1980) 180-day subchronic oral dosing study with resmethrin in Beagle dogs, Waverly, New York, Food and Drug Research Laboratories, 86 pp (Report No. 6289) (Unpublished proprietary data supplied by Roussel Uclaf).

GLICKMAN, A.H. & CASIDA, J.E., (1982) Species and structural variations affecting pyrethroid neurotoxicity. Neurobehav. Toxicol. Teratol., 4: 793-799.

GLOMOT, R. (undated) Etude de la toxicité chronique de 3 semaines chez le rat du RU11484 (NRDC 107) (Unpublished data of Roussel Uclaf submitted to WHO by Wellcome Foundation Ltd).

GLOMOT, R. & CHEVALLIER, B. (1969) Etude de la toxicité aiguë du RU11484 (NRDC 107) Romainville, France, Roussel Uclaf (Rapport Toxico 11386) (Unpublished data).

GRAY, A.J., CONNORS, T.A., HOELLINGER, H., & NGUYEN-HOANG-NAM (1980a) Relationship between the pharmacokinetics of intravenous cismethrin and bioresmethrin and their mammalian toxicity. Pestic. Biochem. Physiol., 13: 281-293.

GRAY, A.J., CONNORS, T.A., & RICKARD, J. (1980b) Mechanism of mammalian toxicity of the pyrethroids. In: Littaner, V.Z., Dudai, Y., Silman, I. Teichberg, V.I., & Vogel, Z., ed. Neurotransmitters and their receptors, New York, John Wiley & Sons Ltd, pp. 565-568.

GREEN, W.M. (1977) Acute dermal LD50 toxicity study on technical resmethrin, Moorestown, New Jersey, Bio-Toxicology Laboratory, 8 pp (Unpublished proprietary data supplied by Roussel Uclaf).

HESS, F.G., THOMPSON, S.W., & BECCI, P.J. (1982) A lifetime evaluation of the dietary administration of SBP-1382 to Wistar albino rats/amendment, Waverly, New York, Food and Drug Research Laboratory, 28 pp (Supplemental report No. 5271) (Unpublished proprietary data supplied by Roussel Uclaf).

HILL, E.F., HEATH, R.G., SPANN, J.W., & WILLIAMS, J.D. (1975) Lethal dietary toxicities of environmental pollutants to birds, Washington, DC, US Department of the Interior, Bureau of Sport Fishery and Wildlife, pp. 1-61 (Report No. 191).

HOELLINGER, H., SONNIER, M., GRAY, A.J., CONNORS, T.A., PICHON, J., & NGUYEN-HOANG-NAM (1985) In vitro covalent binding of cismethrin, bioresmethrin and their common alcohol to hepatic proteins. Toxicol. appl. Pharmacol., 77: 11-18.

HOLMSTEAD, R.L., CASIDA, J.E., & RUZO, L.O. (1977) Photochemical reactions of pyrethroid insecticides. In: Elliott, M., ed. Synthetic pyrethroids, Washington, DC, American Chemical Society (ACS Symposium Series, No. 42).

JACKSON, G.C. & HARDY, C.J. (1984) SBP-1382 acute inhalation toxicity in rats 4-hour exposure, Huntingdon, United Kingdom, Huntingdon Research Centre, 24 pp (Report No. SBP 4a/831042) (Unpublished proprietary data supplied by Roussel Uclaf).

KAGAN, U.S., PANSHINA, T.N., & SASINOVITCH, L.M. (1986) [Biochemical effects of sythetic pyrethroid toxic action.] Gig. i Sanit., 1: 7 (in Russian).

KAUFMAN, D.D. (1986) Degradation and movement of cis- and trans-resmethrin in soil, Beltsville, US Department of Agriculture, 36 pp (Unpublished proprietary data supplied by Roussel Uclaf).

KHOLMATOVA, M. (1984) Hygiene and toxicology of Dravin 755 and Isotrine new pesticides used in agriculture, Alma Ata (Résumé of doctorate thesis).

KNICKERBOCKER, M., BECCI, P.J., COX, G.E., & PARENT, R.A. (1980) A lifetime evaluation of the dietary administration of SBP-1382 to Wistar albino rats, Waverly, New York, Food and Drug Research Laboratories, 110 pp (Report No. 5271) (Unpublished proprietary data supplied by Roussel Uclaf).

LAWRENCE, L.J. & CASIDA, J.E. (1982) Pyrethroid toxicology: Mouse intracerebral structure-toxicity relationship. Pestic. Biochem. Physiol., 18: 9-14.

LAWRENCE, L.J. & CASIDA, J.E. (1983) Stereospecific action of pyrethroid insecticides on the gamma-aminobutyric acid receptor-ionophore complex. Science, 221: 1399-1401.

LAWRENCE, L.J., GEE, K.W., & YAMAMURA, H.I. (1985) Interactions of pyrethroid insecticides with chloride ionophore-associated binding sites. Neurotoxicology, 6: 87-98.

LEAHEY, J.P. (1985) The pyrethroid insecticides, London, Taylor and Francis Ltd, 440 pp.

LUND, A.E. & NARAHASHI, T. (1983) Kinetics of sodium channel modification as the basis for the variation in the nerve membrane effects of pyrethroids and DDT analogs. Pestic. Biochem. Physiol., 20: 203-216.

MACHI, R.A., KAM, C., GALLO, M.A., STEVENS, K.R., & GAGLIARDI, J.J. (1979) Teratological evaluation of SBP-1382 technical in the albino rat, Florham Park, New Jersey, Booz, Allen & Hamilton, Inc., 44 pp (Report No. 2054-066) (Unpublished proprietary data supplied by Roussel Uclaf).

MACKO, J.A., HARVEY, J.G., POPE, C.R., & MCCREESH, A.H. (1979) Hazard evaluation of aerosol formulations containing the synthetic pyrethroid insecticide resmethrin, (5-benzyl-1,3-furyl)methyl-2,2-dimethyl-3-(2-methylpropenyl)cyclopropane-carboxylate (SBP-1382), Aberdeen Proving Ground, US Army Environmental Hygiene Agency, 38 pp (Report No. 75-51-0848-79).

MALONE, J.C. & CHESHER, B.C. (1970) Toxicity to dogs of NRDC 107, Berkhamsted, Wellcome Foundation Ltd (Report No. B 204-70) (Unpublished data).

MARKING, L.L. & MAUCK, W.L. (1975) Toxicity of paired mixtures of candidate forest insecticides to rainbow trout. Bull. environ. Contam. Toxicol., 13: 518-523.

MARTIN, H. & WORTHING, C.R. (1977) The pesticide manual, 5th ed., Croydon, British Crop Protection Council, 461 pp.

MAUCK, W.L., OLSON, L.E., & MARKING, L.L. (1976) Toxicity of natural pyrethroids and five pyrethroids to fish. Arch. environ. Contam. Toxicol., 4: 18-29.

MEISTER, R.T., BERG, G.L., SINE, C., MEISTER, S., & POPLYK, J. (1983) Farm chemical handbook, Section C: Pesticide dictionary, Willoughby, Meister Publishing Co., pp. C205-C206.

MILLER, T.A. & ADAMS, M.E. (1977) Central vs peripheral action of pyrethroids on the housefly nervous system. In: Elliot, M., ed. Synthetic pyrethroids, Washington, DC, American Chemical Society, pp. 98-115 (ACS Symposium Series, No. 42).

MIYAMOTO, J. (1975-76) Terminal residues of bioresmethrin. Submission to IUPAC Terminal Residue Commission, Madrid, September 1975, Leverkusen, September 1976.

MIYAMOTO, J. (1976) Degradation, metabolism and toxicity of synthetic pyrethroids. Environ. Health Perspect., 14: 15-28.

MIYAMOTO, J. (1981) The chemistry metabolism and residue analysis of synthetic pyrethroids. Pure appl. Chem., 53: 1967-2022.

MIYAMOTO, J. & KEARNEY, P.C. (1983) Pesticide chemistry-human welfare and the environment. Proceedings of the Fifth International Congress of Pesticide Chemistry, Kyoto, Japan, 29 August-4 September, 1982, Oxford, Pergamon Press (in 4 volumes).

MIYAMOTO, J., NISHIDA, T., & UEDA, K. (1971) Metabolic fate of resmethrin, 5-benzyl-3-furylmethyl dl-trans-chrysanthemate in the rat. Pestic. Biochem. Physiol., 1: 293-306.

MUMMA, R.O. (1985) Persistence of metabolism of 14C-resmethrin on greenhouse grown tomato fruit, lettuce and field grown wheat, Part III, Pennsylvania State University, 33 pp (Unpublished proprietary data supplied by Roussel Uclaf).

MURANO, A. (1972) Determination of the optical isomers of insecticidal pyrethroids by gas-liquid chromatography. Agric. biol. Chem., 36: 2203-2211.

NIOSH (1983) In: Takten, R.L. & Lewis, R.J., Jr, ed. Registry of toxic effects of chemical substances, 1981-82 edition, Cincinnati, Ohio, National Institute for Occupational Safety and Health, 3057 pp (in 3 volumes).

NISHIUCHI, Y. (1981) [Toxicity of pesticides to some aquatic organisms. I. Toxicity of pesticides to some aquatic insects.] Seitai-Kagaku, 4: 31-46 (in Japanese).

NISHIUCHI, Y. (1982) [Toxicity of pesticides to fish.] Kongetsuno-Noyaku, 26: 105-110 (in Japanese).

NOEL, P.R.B., RIVETT, K.F., CHESTERMAN, H., STREET, A.E., & SPICER, E.J.F. (1971) Oral toxicity study in Beagle dogs (repeated dosage for 3 months), 76 pp (Report No. 3900/71/58) (Unpublished data of Huntingdon Research Centre, United Kingdom).

NORWOOD, T.E. (1986) Preliminary statistical report on assessment of the effects of SBP-1382 40MF (resmethrin) and Scourge (18% resmethrin plus 54% piperonyl butoxide) on non target, aquatic organisms when used for adult mosquito control: results of a field validation study in fresh water ponds in Minnesota, Summer 1984, North Oaks, Minnesota, Mosquito Control Technology, 20 pp (Unpublished proprietary data supplied by Roussel Uclaf).

PIERCE, R.H. (1986) Acute toxicity of Scourge on select estuarine organisms during field applications, Sarasota, Florida, Mote Marine Laboratory, 16 pp (Unpublished proprietary data supplied by Roussel Uclaf).

PLUIJMEN, M., DREVON, C., MONTESANO, R., MALAVEILLE, C., HAUTEFEUILLE, A., & BARTSCH, H. (1984) Lack of mutagenicity of synthetic pyrethroids in *Salmonella typhimurium* strains and in V79 Chinese hamster cells. Mutat. Res., 137: 7-15.

PUCHALSKI, R. (1983) Water solubility and octanol/water partition coefficients of SBP-1382, Lyndhurst, New Jersey, Penick Corporation, 5 pp (Unpublished proprietary data supplied by Roussel Uclaf).

REAGEN, E.L. & BECCI, P.J. (1985a) Acute oral LD50 study of D-L-cis-trans-chrysanthemic acid in Sprague-Dawley rats, Waverly, New York, Food and Drug Research Laboratories, 10 pp (Report No. 8350A) (Unpublished proprietary data supplied by Roussel Uclaf).

REAGEN, E.L. & BECCI, P.J. (1985b) Acute oral LD50 study of D-L-trans-chrysanthemic acid in Sprague-Dawley rats, Waverly, New York, Food and Drug Research Laboratories, 10 pp (Report No. 8350B) (Unpublished proprietary data supplied by Roussel Uclaf).

REAGEN, E.L. & BECCI, P.J. (1985c) Acute oral LD50 study of D-trans-chrysanthemic acid in Sprague-Dawley rats, Waverly, New York, Food and Drug Research Laboratories, 10 pp (Report No. 8350C) (Unpublished proprietary data supplied by Roussel Uclaf).

REAGEN, E.L. & BECCI, P.J. (1985d) Acute oral LD50 study of BFCA 99.6% Sprague-Dawley rats, Waverly, New York, Food and Drug Research Laboratories, 10 pp (Report No. 8725A) (Unpublished proprietary data supplied by Roussel Uclaf).

RIDLEN, R.L., CHRISTOPHER, R.J., WAYNE IRVIE, G., BEIER, R.C., & CAMP, B.J. (1984) Distribution and metabolism of cis and trans-resmethrin in lactating Jersey cows. J. agric. food Chem., 32: 1211-1217.

ROBERTS, N.L., FAIRLEY, C., ANDERSON, A., DAWE, S., & CHANTER, D.O. (1985a) The effects of dietary inclusion of resmethrin on reproduction in the bobwhite quail, Huntingdon, United Kingdom, Huntingdon Research Centre, 34 pp (Report No. SBP 8BT/85957) (Unpublished proprietary data supplied by Roussel Uclaf).

ROBERTS, N.L., FAIRLEY, C., ANDERSON, A., DAWE, S., & CHANTER, D.O. (1985b) The effects of dietary inclusion of resmethrin on reproduction in the mallard duck, Huntingdon, United Kingdom, Huntingdon Research Centre, 28 pp (Report No. SBP 7BT/85550) (Unpublished proprietary data supplied by Roussel Uclaf).

ROPER, E.M. & WRIGHT, G.C. (1984) Sampling efficiency of five solid sorbents for trapping airborne pesticides. Bull. environ. Contam. Toxicol., 33: 476-483.

ROSE, G.P. & DEWAR, A.J. (1983) Intoxication with four synthetic pyrethroids fail to show any correlation between neuromuscular dysfunction and neurobiochemical abnormalities in rats. Arch. Toxicol., 53: 297-316.

RUIGT, G.S.F. & VAN DEN BERCKEN, J. (1986) Action of pyrethroids on a nerve-muscle preparation of the clawed frog, Xenopus laevis. Pestic. Biochem. Physiol., 25: 176-187.

SCHWARTZ, C.S., BECCI, P.J., & PARENT, R.A. (1979a) Evaluation of the neurotoxic effects of SBP-1382 in albino rats. Phase I, Waverly, New York, Food and Drug Research Laboratories, 18 pp (Report No. 6067) (Unpublished proprietary data supplied by Roussel Uclaf).

SCHWARTZ, C.S., BECCI, P.J., & PARENT, R.A. (1979b) Evaluation of the neurotoxic effects of SBP-1382 in albino rats. Phase II, Waverly, New York, Food and Drug Research Laboratories, 17 pp (Report No. 6068) (Unpublished proprietary data supplied by Roussel Uclaf).

SCHWARTZ, C.S., GEPHART, L., BECCI, P.J., & PARENT R.A. (1979c) The evaluation of the effects of SBP-1382 following dietary administration through three generations in Sprague-Dawley rats, Waverly, New York, Food and Drug Research Laboratories, 70 pp (Report No. 5739) (Unpublished proprietary data supplied by Roussel Uclaf).

SEABER, J.A. (1985) Delayed contact hypersensitivity in the guinea pig with SBP-1382 insecticide, Huntingdon, United Kingdom, Huntingdon Research Centre, 14 pp (Report No. 84936D/SBP 10/ss) (Unpublished proprietary data supplied by Roussel Uclaf).

SIMONAITIS, R.A. & CAIL, R.S. (1975) Gas-liquid chromatographic determination of resmethrin in corn, cornmeal, flour, and wheat. J. Assoc. Off. Anal. Chem., 58: 1032-1036.

SJOGREN, R.D. (1985) Assessment of the effects of SBP-1382 40MF (resmethrin) and Scourge (18% resmethrin plus 54% piperonyl butoxide) on non target, aquatic organisms when used for adult mosquito control: results of a field validation study in fresh water ponds in Minnesota, Summer 1984, North Oaks, Minnesota, Mosquito Control Technology, 105 pp (Unpublished proprietary data supplied by Roussel Uclaf).

SMITH, P.R. (1980) The effect of cismethrin on the rat dorsal root potentials. Eur. J. Pharmacol., 66: 125-128.

STAUFFER (1984) Ethyl chrysanthemate/Product safety informaton, Westport, USA, Stauffer Chemical Co., 5 pp.

SWENTZEL, K.L., ANGERHOFER, R.A., & HAIGHT, E.A. (1977) Toxicological evaluation of pyrethroid insecticide (5-benzyl-1,3-furyl)methyl-2,2-dimethyl-3-(2-methylpropenyl)cyclopropanecarboxylate (resmethrin), Aberdeen Proving Ground, US Army Environmental Hygiene Agency (Report No. 51-0830-77).

UEDA, K., GAUGHAN, L.C., & CASIDA, J.E. (1974) Photodecomposition of resmethrin and related pyrethroids. J. agric. food Chem., 22: 212-220.

UEDA, K., GAUGHAN, L.C., & CASIDA, J.E. (1975a) Metabolism of four resmethrin isomers by liver microsomes. Pestic. Biochem. Physiol., 5: 280-294.

UEDA, K., GAUGHAN, L.C., & CASIDA, J.E. (1975b) Metabolism of (+)-trans- and (+)-cis-resmethrin in rats. J. agric. food Chem., 23: 106-115.

UNO, M., OKADA, T., OHMAE, T., & TANIGAWA, K. (1982) [Determination of pyrethroid insecticides by dual-wavelength densitometry.] Shokuhin Eiseigaku Zasshi, 23: 191-195 (in Japanese).

US ENVIRONMENTAL PROTECTION AGENCY (1983) Tolerances for pesticides in food administered by EPA: Resmethrin. Fed. Reg., 48: 36246-36247.

VAN DEN BERCKEN, J. (1977) The action of allethrin on the peripheral nervous system of the frog. Pestic. Sci., 8: 692-699.

VAN DEN BERCKEN, J. & VIJVERBERG, H.P.M. (1980) Voltage clamp studies on the effects of allethrin and DDT on the sodium channels in frog myelinated nerve membrane. In: Insect neurobiology and pesticide action, London, Society of Chemical Industry, pp. 79-85.

VAN DEN BERCKEN, J., AKKERMANS, L.M.A., & VAN DER ZALM, J.M. (1973) DDT-likeaction of allethrin in the sensory nervous system of Xenopus laevis. Eur. J. Pharmacol., 21: 95-106.

VAN DEN BERCKEN, J., KROESE, A.B.A., & AKKERMANS, L.M.A. (1979) Effect of insecticides on the sensory nervous system. In: Narahashi, T., ed. Neurotoxicology of insecticides and pheromones, New York, London, Plenum Press, pp. 182-210.

VANNIER, B. & FOURNEX, R. (1986) Bioresmethrin. Detection of a mutagenic potency (micronucleus test in the mouse), Romainville, France, Roussel Uclaf, 16 pp (Report No. RU-BRM-85612-BB/178/A) (Unpublished proprietary data).

VERSCHOYLE, R.D. & ALDRIDGE, W.N. (1980) Structure-activity relationship of some pyrethroids in rats. Arch. Toxicol., 45: 325-329.

VERSCHOYLE, R.D. & BARNES, J.M. (1972) Toxicity of natural and synthetic pyrethrins in rats. Pestic. Biochem. Physiol., 2(3): 308-311.

VIJVERBERG, H.P.M. & VAN DEN BERCKEN, J. (1979) Frequency dependent effects of the pyrethroid insecticide decamethrin in frog myelinated nerve fibres. Eur. J. Pharmacol., 58: 501-504.

VIJVERBERG, H.P.M. & VAN DEN BERCKEN, J. (1982) Action of pyrethroid insecticides on the vertebrate nervous system. Neuropathol. appl. Neurobiol., 8: 421-440.

VIJVERBERG, H.P.M., RUIGT, G.S.F., & VAN DEN BERCKEN, J. (1982a) Structure-related effects of pyrethroid insecticides on the lateral-line sense organ and on peripheral nerves of the clawed frog, Xenopus laevis. Pestic. Biochem. Physiol., 18: 315-324.

VIJVERBERG, H.P.M., VAN DER ZALM, J.M., & VAN DEN BERCKEN, J. (1982b) Similar mode of action of pyrethroids and DDT on sodium channel gating in myelinated nerves. Nature (Lond.), 295: 601-603.

VIJVERBERG, H.P.M., VAN DER ZALM, J.M., VAN KLEEF, R.G.D.M., & VAN DEN BERCKEN, J. (1983) Temperature and structure-dependent interaction of pyrethroids with the sodium channels in frog node of Ranvier. Biochim. Biophys. Acta, 728: 73-82.

VOLKOV, U.P., STRELETS, I.P., & TIULENEV, K.L. (1979) [Progress in the field of pyrethroids and their synergists. Collection of articles on household chemistry.] Moscow, Volume 7, p. 125 (in Russian).

WALDRON, M.M. (1969) Foetal toxicity study - 95 H 56 - given orally in the rabbit (Report Path 51) (Unpublished data of Wellcome Foundation Ltd).

WALLWORK, L.M. & MALONE, J.C. (1971) Potentiation toxicity studies with NRDC 107, bioallethrin and piperonyl butoxide (Report No. B 47-71) (Unpublished data of Wellcome Foundation Ltd).

WALLWORK, L.M. & MALONE, J.C. (1972) Bioresmethrin. Preliminary 24 hour rat inhalation study (Report No. B 290-72) (Unpublished data of Wellcome Foundation Ltd).

WALLWORK, L.M., CHESHER, B.C., & MALONE J.C. (1970) Toxicity of NRDC 107 to laboratory animals (Report No. B 199-70) (Unpublished data of Wellcome Foundation Ltd).

WALLWORK, L.M., CLAMPITT, R.B., & MALONE, J.C. (1971) NRDC 107, rat oral 91 day toxicity study (Report No. B 199-71) (Unpublished data of Wellcome Foundation Ltd).

WATSON, S.C. (1984) Photolysis study of SBP-1382 resmethrin (final report), Columbus, Ohio, Battelle Columbus Laboratory, 10 pp (Unpublished proprietary data supplied by Roussel Uclaf).

WEEKS, M.H., LELAND, T.M., BOLDT, R.E., MELLICK, P.W., & STEINBERG, M. (1972) Toxicological evaluation of pyrethroid insecticide (5-benzyl-3-furyl) methyl-2,2-dimethyl-3-(2-methylpropenyl) cyclopropanecarboxylate (SBP-1382), Aberdeen Proving Ground, US Army Environmental Hygiene Agency, 44 pp (Special study No. 51-127-71/72).

WHITE, I.N.H., VERSCHOYLE, R.D., MORADIAN, M.H., & BARNES, J.M. (1976) The relationship between brain levels of cismethrin and bioresmethrin in female rats and neurotoxic effects. Pestic. Biochem. Physiol., 6: 491-500.

WHO (1979) WHO Technical Report Series, No. 634 (Safe use of pesticides. Third Report of the WHO Expert Committee on Vector Biology and Control), pp. 18-23.

WHO (1986) The WHO recommended classification of pesticides by hazard and guidelines to classification 1986-1987, Geneva, World Health Organization, p. 38 (VBC/86.1, Rev. 1).

WHO/FAO (1978) Data sheet on pesticides No. 34: Bioresmethrin, Geneva, World Health Organization (WHO/VBC/DS/78.34).

WORTHING, C.R. & WALKER, S.B. (1983) The pesticide manual, 7th ed., Croydon, British Crop Protection Council, 485 pp.

WOUTERS, W. & VAN DEN BERCKEN, J. (1978) Action of pyrethroids. Gen. Pharmacol., 9: 387-398.

YOSHIOKA, H. (1980) [Chemistry and action of the recent synthetic pyrethroids and their stereoisomers.] J. synth. org. Chem. Japan, 38: 1151-1162 (in Japanese).

APPENDIX

On the basis of electrophysiological studies with peripheral nerve preparations of frogs (Xenopus laevis; Rana temporaria, and Rana esculenta), it is possible to distinguish between 2 classes of pyrethroid insecticides: (Type I and Type II). A similar distinction between these 2 classes of pyrethroids has been made on the basis of the symptoms of toxicity in mammals and insects (Van den Bercken et al., 1979; WHO, 1979; Verschoyle & Aldridge, 1980; Glickman & Casida, 1982; Lawrence & Casida, 1982). The same distinction was found in studies on cockroaches by Gammon et al. (1981).

Based on the binding assay on the gamma-aminobutyric acid (GABA) receptor-ionophore complex, synthetic pyrethroids can also be classified into two types: the α-cyano-3-phenoxybenzyl pyrethroids and the non-cyano pyrethroids (Gammon et al., 1982; Gammon & Casida, 1983; Lawrence & Casida, 1983; Lawrence et al., 1985).

Pyrethroids that do not contain an α-cyano group (allethrin, d-phenothrin, permethrin, tetramethrin, cismethrin, and bioresmethrin) (Type I: T-syndrome)

The pyrethroids that do not contain an α-cyano group give rise to pronounced repetitive activity in sense organs and in sensory nerve fibres (Van den Bercken et al., 1973). At room temperature, this repetitive activity usually consists of trains of 3-10 impulses and occasionally up to 25 impulses. Train duration is between 10 and 5 milliseconds.

These compounds also induce pronounced repetitive firing of the presynaptic motor nerve terminal in the neuromuscular junction (Van den Bercken, 1977). There was no significant effect of the insecticide on neurotransmitter release or on the sensitivity of the subsynaptic membrane or the muscle fibre membrane. Presynaptic repetitive firing was also observed in the sympathetic ganglion treated with these pyrethroids.

In the lateral-line sense organ and in the motor nerve terminal, but not in the cutaneous touch receptor or in sensory nerve fibres, the pyrethroid-induced repetitive activity increases dramatically as the temperature is lowered, and a decrease of 5 °C in temperature may cause a more than 3-fold increase in the number of repetitive impulses per train. This effect is easily reversed by raising the temperature. The origin of this "negative temperature coefficient" is not clear (Vijverberg et al., 1983).

Synthetic pyrethroids act directly on the axon through interference with the sodium channel gating mechanism that underlies the generation and conduction of each nerve impulse. The transitional state of the sodium channel is controlled by 2 separately acting gating mechanisms, referred to as the activation gate and the inactivation gate. Since pyrethroids only appear to affect the sodium current during depolarization, the rapid opening of the activation gate and the slow closing of the inactivation gate proceed normally. However, once the sodium channel is open, the activation gate is restrained in the open position by the pyrethroid molecule. While all pyrethroids have essentially the same basic mechanism of action, the rate of relaxation differs substantially for the various pyrethroids (Flannigan & Tucker, 1985).

In the isolated node of Ranvier, allethrin causes prolongation of the transient increase in sodium permeability of the nerve membrane during excitation (Van den Bercken & Vijverberg, 1980). Evidence so far available indicates that allethrin selectively slows down the closing of the activation gate of a fraction of the sodium channels that open during depolarization of the membrane. The time constant of closing of the activation gate in the allethrin-affected channels is about 100 milliseconds compared with less than 100 microseconds in the normal sodium channel, i.e., it is slowed down by a factor of more than 100. This results in a marked prolongation of the sodium current across the nerve membrane during excitation, and this prolonged sodium current is directly responsible for the repetitive activity induced by allethrin (Vijverberg et al., 1983).

The effects of cismethrin on synaptic transmission in the frog neuromuscular junction, as reported by Evans (1976), are almost identical to those of allethrin, i.e., presynaptic repetitive firing, and no significant effects on transmitter release or on the subsynaptic membrane.

Interestingly, the action of these pyrethroids closely resembles that of the insecticide DDT in the peripheral nervous system of the frog. DDT also causes pronounced repetitive activity in sense organs, in sensory nerve fibres, and in motor nerve terminals, due to a prolongation of the transient increase in sodium permeability of the nerve membrane during excitation. Recently, it was demonstrated that allethrin and DDT have essentially the same effect on sodium channels in frog myelinated nerve membrane. Both compounds slow down the rate of closing of a fraction of the sodium channels that open on depolarization of the membrane (Van den Bercken et al., 1973, 1979; Vijverberg et al., 1982b).

In the electrophysiological experiments using giant axons of crayfish, the Type I pyrethroids and DDT analogues retain sodium channels in a modified open state only intermittently, cause large depolarizing afterpotentials, and evoke repetitive firing with minimal effect on the resting potential (Lund & Narahashi, 1983).

These results strongly suggest that permethrin and cismethrin, like allethrin, primarily affect the sodium channels in the nerve membrane and cause a prolongation of the transient increase in sodium permeability of the membrane during excitation.

The effects of pyrethroids on end-plate and muscle action potentials were studied in the pectoralis nerve-muscle preparation of the clawed frog (Xenopus laevis). Type I pyrethroids (allethrin, cismethrin, bioresmethrin, and 1R, cis-phenothrin) caused moderate presynaptic repetitive activity, resulting in the occurrence of multiple end-plate potentials (Ruigt & Van den Bercken, 1986).

Pyrethroids with an α-cyano group on the 3-phenoxybenzyl alcohol (deltamethrin, cypermethrin, fenvalerate, and fenpropanate) (Type II: CS-syndrome)

The pyrethroids with an α-cyano group cause an intense repetitive activity in the lateral-line organ in the form of long-lasting trains of impulses (Vijverberg et al., 1982a). Such a train may last for up to 1 min and contains thousands of impulses. The duration of the trains and the number of impulses per train increase markedly on lowering the temperature. Cypermethrin does not cause repetitive activity in myelinated nerve fibres. Instead, this pyrethroid causes a frequency-dependent depression of the nervous impulse, brought about by a progressive depolarization of the nerve membrane as a result of the summation of depolarizing after-potentials during train stimulation (Vijverberg & Van den Bercken, 1979; Vijverberg et al., 1983).

In the isolated node of Ranvier, cypermethrin, like allethrin, specifically affects the sodium channels of the nerve membrane and causes a long-lasting prolongation of the transient increase in sodium permeability during excitation, presumably by slowing down the closing of the activation gate of the sodium channel (Vijverberg & Van den Bercken, 1979; Vijverberg et al., 1983). The time constant of closing of the activation gate in the cypermethrin-affected channels is prolonged to more than 100 milliseconds. Apparently, the amplitude of the prolonged sodium current after cypermethrin is too small to induce repetitive activity in nerve fibres, but is sufficient to cause the long-lasting repetitive firing in the lateral-line sense organ.

These results suggest that α-cyano pyrethroids primarily affect the sodium channels in the nerve membrane and cause a long-lasting prolongation of the transient increase in sodium permeability of the membrane during excitation.

In the electrophysiological experiments using giant axons of crayfish, the Type II pyrethroids retain sodium channels in a modified continuous open state persistently, depolarize the membrane, and block the action potential without causing repetitive firing (Lund & Narahashi, 1983).

Diazepam, which facilitates GABA reaction, delayed the onset of action of deltamethrin and fenvalerate, but not permethrin and allethrin, in both the mouse and cockroach. Possible mechanisms of the Type II pyrethroid syndrome include action at the GABA receptor complex or a closely linked class of neuroreceptor (Gammon et al., 1982).

The Type II syndrome of intracerebrally administered pyrethroids closely approximates that of the convulsant picrotoxin (PTX). Deltamethrin inhibits the binding of [^{3}H]-dihydropicrotoxin to rat brain synaptic membranes, whereas the non-toxic R epimer of deltamethrin is inactive. These findings suggest a possible relation between the Type II pyrethroid action and the GABA receptor complex. The stereospecific correlation between the toxicity of Type II pyrethroids and their potency to inhibit the [^{35}S]-TBPS binding was established using a radioligand, [^{35}S]-*t*-butylbicyclophosphoro-thionate [^{35}S]-TBPS. Studies with 37 pyrethroids revealed an absolute correlation, without any false positive or negative, between mouse intracerebral toxicity and *in vitro* inhibition: all toxic cyano compounds including deltamethrin, [1R,*cis*]-cypermethrin, [1R,*trans*]-cypermethrin, and [2S, αS]-fenvalerate were inhibitors, but their non-toxic stereoisomers were not; non-cyano pyrethroids were much less potent or were inactive (Lawrence & Casida, 1983).

In the [^{35}S]-TBPS and [^{3}H]-Ro 5-4864 (a convulsant benzodiazepine radioligand) binding assay, the inhibitory potencies of pyrethroids were closely related to their mammalian toxicities. The most toxic pyrethroids of Type II were the most potent inhibitors of [^{3}H]-Ro 5-4864 specific binding to rat brain membranes. The [^{3}H]-dihydropicrotoxin and [^{35}S]-TBPS binding studies with pyrethroids strongly indicated that Type II effects of pyrethroids are mediated, at least in part, through an interaction with a GABA-regulated chloride ionophore-associated binding site. Moreover, studies with [^{3}H]-Ro 5-4864 support this hypothesis and, in addition, indicate that the pyrethroid-binding site may be very closely related to the convulsant benzodiazepine site of action (Lawrence et al., 1985).

The Type II pyrethroids (deltamethrin, [1R,*cis*]-cypermethrin and [2S,αS]-fenvalerate) increased the input resistance of crayfish claw opener muscle fibres bathed in GABA. In contrast, two non-insecticidal stereoisomers and Type I pyrethroids (permethrin, resmethrin, allethrin) were inactive. Therefore, cyanophenoxybenzyl pyrethroids appear to act on the GABA receptor-ionophore complex (Gammon & Casida, 1983).

The effects of pyrethroids on end-plate and muscle action potentials were studied in the pectoralis nerve-muscle preparation of the clawed frog (Xenopus laevis). Type II pyrethroids (cypermethrin and deltamethrin) induced trains of repetitive muscle action potentials without presynaptic repetitive activity. However, an intermediate group of pyrethroids (1R-permethrin, cyphenothrin, and fenvalerate) caused both types of effect. Thus, in muscle or nerve membrane the pyrethroid induced repetitive activities due to a prolongation of the sodium current. But no clear distinction was observed between non-cyano and α-cyano pyrethroids (Ruigt & Van den Bercken, 1986).

Appraisal

In summary, the results strongly suggest that the primary target site of pyrethroid insecticides in the vertebrate nervous system is the sodium channel in the nerve membrane. Pyrethroids without an α-cyano group (allethrin, d-phenothrin, permethrin, and cismethrin) cause a moderate prolongation of the transient increase in sodium permeability of the nerve membrane during excitation. This results in relatively short trains of repetitive nerve impulses in sense organs, sensory (afferent) nerve fibres, and, in effect, nerve terminals. On the other hand, the α-cyano pyrethroids cause a long-lasting prolongation of the transient increase in sodium permeability of the nerve membrane during excitation. This results in long-lasting trains of repetitive impulses in sense organs and a frequency-dependent depression of the nerve impulse in nerve fibres. The difference in effects between permethrin and cypermethrin, which have identical molecular structures except for the presence of an α-cyano group on the phenoxybenzyl alcohol, indicates that it is this α-cyano group that is responsible for the long-lasting prolongation of the sodium permeability.

Since the mechanisms responsible for nerve impulse generation and conduction are basically the same throughout the entire nervous system, pyrethroids may also induce repetitive activity in various parts of the brain. The difference in symptoms of poisoning by α-cyano pyrethroids, compared with the classical pyrethroids, is not necessarily due to an exclusive central site of action. It may be related to the long-lasting repetitive activity in sense organs and possibly in other parts of the nervous system, which, in a more advance state of poisoning, may be accompanied by a frequency-dependent depression of the nervous impulse.

Pyrethroids also cause pronounced repetitive activity and a prolongation of the transient increase in sodium permeability of the nerve membrane in insects and other invertebrates. Available information indicates that the sodium channel in the nerve membrane is also the most important target site of pyrethroids in the invertebrate nervous system (Wouters & Van den Bercken, 1978; WHO, 1979).

Because of the universal character of the processes underlying nerve excitability, the action of pyrethroids should not be considered restricted to particular animal species, or to a certain region of the nervous system. Although it has been established that sense organs and nerve endings are the most vulnerable to the action of pyrethroids, the ultimate lesion that causes death will depend on the animal species, environmental conditions, and on the chemical structure and physical characteristics of the pyrethroid molecule (Vijverberg & Van den Bercken, 1982).

Other titles available in the ENVIRONMENTAL HEALTH CRITERIA series (continued):

67. Tetradifon
68. Hydrazine
69. Magnetic Fields
70. Principles for the Safety Assessment of Food Additives and Contaminants in Food
71. Pentachlorophenol
72. Principles of Studies on Diseases of Suspected Chemical Etiology and Their Prevention
73. Phosphine and Selected Metal Phosphides
74. Diaminotoluenes
75. Toluene Diisocyanates
76. Thiocarbamate Pesticides — A General Introduction
77. Man-Made Mineral Fibres
78. Dithiocarbamate Pesticides, Ethylenethiourea, and Propylenethiourea — A General Introduction
79. Dichlorvos
80. Pyrrolizidine Alkaloids
81. Vanadium
82. Cypermethrin
83. DDT and its Derivatives — Environmental Aspects
84. 2,4-Dichlorophenoxyacetic Acid — Environmental Aspects
85. Lead — Environmental Aspects
86. Mercury — Environmental Aspects
87. Allethrins
88. Polychlorinated Dibenzo-*para*-dioxins and Dibenzofurans
89. Formaldehyde
90. Dimethoate
91. Aldrin and Dieldrin